T0252103

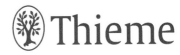

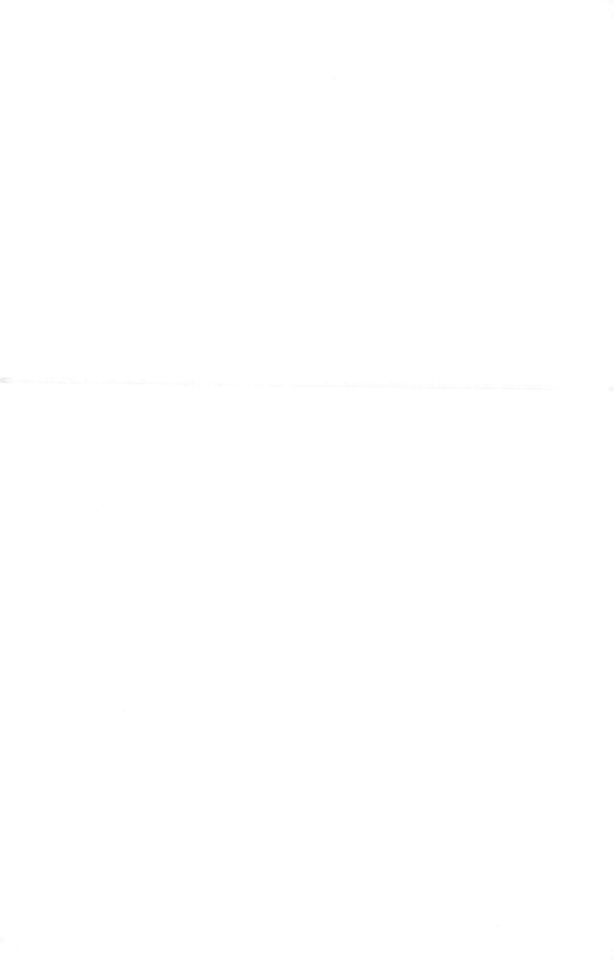

Ultrasound Q&A Review for the Boards

Adrian Dawkins, MD
Chief, Division of Abdominal Radiology
Medical Director of Radiology
Associate Professor
Department of Radiology
University of Kentucky
Lexington, Kentucky

236 illustrations

Thieme
New York • Stuttgart • Delhi • Rio de Janeiro

Library of Congress Cataloging-in-Publication Data is available from the publisher

Important note: Medicine is an ever-changing science undergoing continual development. Research and clinical experience are continually expanding our knowledge, in particular our knowledge of proper treatment and drug therapy. Insofar as this book mentions any dosage or application, readers may rest assured that the authors, editors, and publishers have made every effort to ensure that such references are in accordance with **the state of knowledge at the time of production of the book.**

Nevertheless, this does not involve, imply, or express any guarantee or responsibility on the part of the publishers in respect to any dosage instructions and forms of applications stated in the book. **Every user is requested to examine carefully** the manufacturers' leaflets accompanying each drug and to check, if necessary in consultation with a physician or specialist, whether the dosage schedules mentioned therein or the contraindications stated by the manufacturers differ from the statements made in the present book. Such examination is particularly important with drugs that are either rarely used or have been newly released on the market. Every dosage schedule or every form of application used is entirely at the user's own risk and responsibility. The authors and publishers request every user to report to the publishers any discrepancies or inaccuracies noticed. If errors in this work are found after publication, errata will be posted at www.thieme.com on the product description page.

Some of the product names, patents, and registered designs referred to in this book are in fact registered trademarks or proprietary names even though specific reference to this fact is not always made in the text. Therefore, the appearance of a name without designation as proprietary is not to be construed as a representation by the publisher that it is in the public domain.

©2020. Thieme. All rights reserved.

Thieme Publishers New York
333 Seventh Avenue, New York, NY 10001 USA
+1 800 782 3488, customerservice@thieme.com

Georg Thieme Verlag KG
Rüdigerstrasse 14, 70469 Stuttgart, Germany
+49 [0]711 8931 421, customerservice@thieme.de

Thieme Publishers Delhi
A-12, Second Floor, Sector-2, Noida-201301
Uttar Pradesh, India
+91 120 45 566 00, customerservice@thieme.in

Thieme Publishers Rio de Janeiro,
Thieme Publicações Ltda.
Edifício Rodolpho de Paoli, 25° andar
Av. Nilo Peçanha, 50 – Sala 2508,
Rio de Janeiro 20020-906 Brasil
+55 21 3172-2297

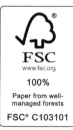

FSC
www.fsc.org
100%
Paper from well-managed forests
FSC® C103101

Cover design: Thieme Publishing Group
Typesetting by Thomson Digital, India

Printed in USA by King Printing Company, Inc.   5 4 3 2 1

ISBN 978-1-62623-485-7

Also available as an e-book:
eISBN 978-1-62623-486-4

To my loving wife, Nanditha, and my sons, Zayden and Kiyan. Without your love and support this book would not exist.

To my mother, Cynthia. Thank you for creating the foundation.

Adrian Dawkins

Contents

Preface

I am constantly in awe of ultrasound technology. I have been fortunate to witness the practice of ultrasound by talented radiologists on both sides of the "pond". As a young resident (registrar) in the north of England, I was able to observe and practice ultrasound in its purest form: a clinical question addressed by a physician with a transducer in hand. This was tremendously insightful, fostering an appreciation for the technical skill and medical knowledge that need to coexist. The high volume environment of a busy American medical center provided ample opportunity to learn from seasoned and nationally recognized experts as they interacted with highly skilled sonographers to make accurate and timely diagnoses. These experiences created the foundation for the manner in which I practice ultrasound.

It wouldn't be an exaggeration to say that the practice of ultrasound is changing tremendously from month to month. The advent of point of care ultrasound (POCUS) has brought ultrasound within the reach of many medical practitioners. Radiology training programs need to ensure adequate ultrasound training for residents if future radiologists are to remain relevant in ultrasound practice. Currently, ultrasound remains one of the 18 categories tested within the American Board of Radiology's "Core" examination.

In this book, we present a series of questions to guide radiology trainees as they prepare to undertake their board examinations. The book is generally arranged in an organ-based approach and questions are inspired by everyday practice. The purpose of writing this book is to present easy-to-understand cases to aid recall and to reinforce common ultrasound concepts. We have also included a chapter on physics to provide a more comprehensive review. References are provided at the end of each chapter, should the reader require further information. My coauthors are very knowledgeable in various aspects of ultrasound. My appreciation extends to all the coauthors for generously contributing chapters to this book. We hope that this offering will be deemed useful for radiology trainees, imparting some of the knowledge that we have gained through years of medical practice.

Adrian Dawkins, MD

Acknowledgments

I would like to thank Dr. Kimberly Absher, Assistant Professor of Pathology and Laboratory Medicine, University of Kentucky; Dr. Scott Berl, Radiologist, Jackson Imaging Center, Jackson Hospital, Montgomery Alabama; Dr. Gerald Broussard, Radiologist, Comprehensive Radiology Services, Mississippi; and Dr. Riham El Khouli, Assistant Professor of Radiology, University of Kentucky, without whom this book would not have been possible.

Adrian Dawkins, MD

Contributors

Adrian Dawkins, MD
Chief, Division of Abdominal Radiology
Medical Director of Radiology
Associate Professor
Department of Radiology
University of Kentucky
Lexington, Kentucky

Halemane Ganesh, MD
Assistant Professor
Department of Radiology
University of Kentucky
Lexington, Kentucky

Gary Ge, MS
Medical Physicist
Department of Radiology
VA Medical Center
Lexington, Kentucky

Nanditha George, MD
Staff Radiologist
Appalachian Regional Healthcare, Medical Mall
Hazard, Kentucky

Karen Tran-Harding, MD
Abdominal Radiology Fellow
Department of Radiological Sciences
University of California
Irvine, California

Rashmi Nair, MD
Assistant Professor
Department of Radiology
University of Kentucky
Lexington, Kentucky

Barbara Pawley, MD
Associate Professor
Department of Radiology
University of Kentucky
Lexington, Kentucky

Edward Richer, MD
Assistant Professor
Department of Radiology
Emory University
Atlanta, Georgia

Paul J. Spicer, MD
Associate Professor
Department of Radiology
University of Kentucky
Lexington, Kentucky

Scott Stevens, MD
Associate Professor
Department of Radiology
University of Kentucky
Lexington, Kentucky

Chapter 1

Gynecology and First Trimester Obstetrics

Adrian Dawkins and Nanditha George

1   Questions and Answers

Question 1.1: The Society of Radiologists in Ultrasound (SRU) Consensus Conference statement, published in *Radiology* in September 2010, addresses adnexal cysts in which group of women?
A. Symptomatic pregnant women.
B. Asymptomatic nonpregnant women.
C. Symptomatic premenopausal women.
D. Asymptomatic postmenopausal women.

Answer:
B. Correct. The SRU Consensus statement addressed lesions in asymptomatic nonpregnant women, both pre- and postmenopausal. While the recommendations may be useful in symptomatic women, the overall clinical picture should help steer management in these patients.

A, C, D—Incorrect. Asymptomatic nonpregnant women are addressed.

Question 1.2: What precise cyst measurement should be used to guide management of adnexal cysts according to the SRU Consensus statement (*Radiology* 2010)?
A. Maximum diameter in the sagittal plane.
B. Maximum diameter in the transverse plane.
C. Mean diameter.
D. Maximum diameter in any plane.

Answer:
D. Correct. The maximum diameter in any plane was chosen, since measurements in all three planes may be altered by pressure created by the endocavitary vaginal transducer.

A, B, C—Incorrect. The maximum diameter in any plane is used.

Question 1.3: These images were obtained in a 28-year-old female with abdominal pain. What is the likely cause for this appearance?

A. Endometriosis.

B. Ovarian hyperstimulation.

C. Molar pregnancy.

D. Ectopic pregnancy.

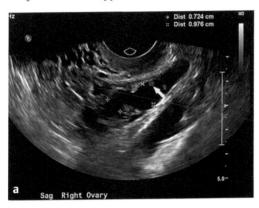

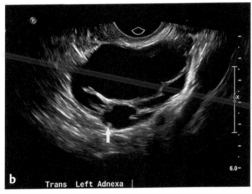

Answer:

A. Correct. The images demonstrate bilateral tubular fluid-filled structures within the adnexa. Also, tiny projections (*arrows*), due to longitudinal folds, can be seen protruding into the lumen. This has been described as the "cogwheel sign" and is typical of hydrosalpinx. Of the choices, endometriosis best explains the presence of bilateral hydrosalpinges.

B. Incorrect. Enlarged ovaries are seen in ovarian hyperstimulation.

C. Incorrect. Enlarged ovaries containing theca lutein cyst may be present in cases of molar pregnancy.

D. Incorrect. An ectopic pregnancy would not typically result in this appearance.

Question 1.4: A 54-year-old postmenopausal female undergoes a pelvic ultrasound due to an incidental left ovarian finding on computed tomography (CT). Which statement regarding management of this finding is correct?

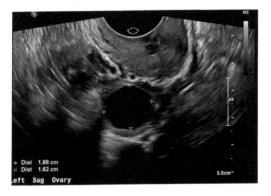

A. No follow-up is required.

B. Follow-up in 1 year is recommended.

C. Pelvic magnetic resonance imaging (MRI) is recommended for better characterization.

D. None of the above.

Answer:

A. Correct. Recently published updated guidelines by the Society of Radiologists in Ultrasound (SRU) suggest that simple cysts in asymptomatic postmenopausal females require no follow-up if less than or equal to 3cm in size.

B. Incorrect. No follow-up is recommended.

C. Incorrect. Pelvic MRI may be of value for larger cysts if deemed to be not well-evaluated with ultrasound.

D. Incorrect. No follow-up is recommended.

Question 1.5: A 25-year-old woman presents with irregular menstrual bleeding and undergoes a pelvic ultrasound. A lesion is found within her right ovary. Which statement is correct?

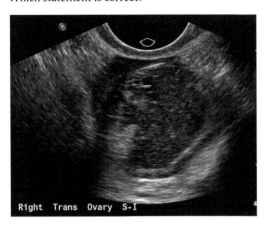

A. The appearance is consistent with an endometrioma.

B. The appearance is consistent with a hemorrhagic cyst.

C. The appearance is consistent with a peritoneal inclusion cyst.

D. The appearance is consistent with a dermoid.

Answer:

D. Correct. The image demonstrates a complex cyst with an echogenic focus within the inferior aspect, toward the left of the image, consistent with fat. Short horizontal dash-like echogenic foci are also noted as well as tiny echogenic dots throughout the lesion. This had been described as the "dot-dash sign." The findings are classic for an ovarian dermoid cyst.

A. Incorrect. An endometrioma is characterized by homogenous low-level echoes.

B. Incorrect. The typical hemorrhagic cyst demonstrates a mesh-like pattern.

C. Incorrect. A peritoneal inclusion cyst is fairly simple in morphology but conforms to the surrounding pelvic structures.

Question 1.6: Which statement best represents the appropriate management of the lesion seen in (Question 1.5)?

A. This lesion should be aspirated and sent for cytologic analysis.

B. A trial of danazol should be initiated.

C. No follow-up is required.

D. Repeat ultrasound in 6 months to 1 year.

Answer:

D. Correct. A dermoid should initially be re-evaluated with follow-up ultrasound in 6 months to 1 year to document stability. There is a very small risk (1%) of malignant transformation albeit in larger dermoids.

A. Incorrect. Aspiration of cystic ovarian lesions is generally avoided since the yield of useful diagnostic material is very low. There is also the risk of peritoneal seeding.

B. Incorrect. Danazol is a synthetic steroid, used to treat endometriosis.

C. Incorrect. A dermoid should initially be re-evaluated with follow-up ultrasound in 6 months to 1 year to document stability.

Question 1.7: Regarding early pregnancy, which statement is correct?

A.   A nonviable pregnancy can be confirmed trans-abdominally if the crown–rump length measures at least 10 mm and no cardiac activity is detected.

B.   A positive serum pregnancy test is defined as a beta human chorionic gonadotropin (HCG) value of 3 mlU/mL and above.

C.   A pregnancy of unknown location is defined as one in which there is a positive serum or urine pregnancy test, with no discernible intrauterine gestational sac or sonographic evidence of an ectopic on a transvaginal scan.

D.   A nonviable pregnancy is defined as one which has not yet reached 26 weeks gestation.

Answer:

C. Correct. A pregnancy of unknown location is defined as one in which there is a positive serum or urine pregnancy test, with no discernible intrauterine gestational sac or sonographic evidence of an ectopic on a transvaginal scan.

A. Incorrect. A nonviable pregnancy can be confirmed transabdominally if the crown–rump length measures at least 15 mm and no cardiac activity is detected.

B. Incorrect. A positive serum pregnancy test is defined as a beta HCG value of 5 mlU/mL and above.

D. Incorrect. A nonviable pregnancy is defined as one which has no chance of resulting in a liveborn child, for example, an ectopic pregnancy.

Question 1.8: A 32-year-old patient presents with sharp left-sided pelvic pain and a positive urine beta HCG. A pelvic ultrasound is performed. Given the sonographic findings and patient symptoms, what is the likelihood of an ectopic pregnancy?

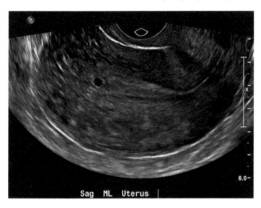

A.   1 in 30,000.
B.   1 in 3,000.
C.   1 in 300.
D.   1 in 30.

Answer:

A. Correct. The image demonstrates the normal appearance of an early intrauterine pregnancy (IUP). The presence of an ectopic pregnancy in conjunction with an IUP, that is a heterotopic pregnancy, is very unlikely occurring in 1 in 30,000 pregnancies.

B, C, D—Incorrect. A heterotopic pregnancy occurs in 1 in 30,000 pregnancies.

Question 1.9: If the image in (Question 1.8) represents a normal early pregnancy, which structure should develop next?
A.   Yolk sac.
B.   Amnion.
C.   Fetal pole.
D.   Gestational sac.

Answer:
A. **Correct.** The yolk sac is the first structure to develop within the gestational sac in a normal pregnancy.

B. Incorrect. The yolk sac is visible before the amnion can be discerned.

C. Incorrect. The yolk sac is visible before the fetal pole can be discerned.

D. Incorrect. The gestational sac is the first sonographically detected structure to develop in a normal pregnancy.

Question 1.10: Regarding this image, which statement is correct?

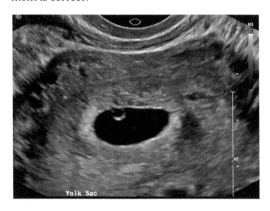

A.   The pregnancy should be dated by the mean gestational sac diameter.
B.   The pregnancy should be dated by the greatest gestational sac diameter.
C.   The pregnancy should be dated by the mean yolk sac diameter.
D.   The pregnancy should be dated by the greatest yolk sac diameter.

Answer:
A. **Correct**. At this point in the pregnancy, the mean diameter of the gestational sac is used to date the pregnancy.

B. Incorrect. The mean diameter of the gestational sac is used to date the pregnancy.

C, D—Incorrect. The size of the yolk sac is not used to date a pregnancy.

Question 1.11: Regarding the image in (Question 1.10), which statement is correct?

A. After 11 days, the absence of an embryo with cardiac activity is diagnostic of pregnancy failure.

B. If the mean sac diameter is 20 mm, the findings are diagnostic of pregnancy failure.

C. The yolk sac develops in the 7th week of pregnancy.

D. A yolk sac diameter of 7 mm is diagnostic of pregnancy failure.

Answer:

A. Correct. After 11 days, the absence of an embryo with cardiac activity is diagnostic of pregnancy failure.

B. Incorrect. A mean sac diameter of 25 mm, in the absence of an embryo is diagnostic of pregnancy failure.

C. Incorrect. The yolk sac develops at 5½ weeks.

D. Incorrect. A yolk sac diameter above 5 mm is highly suggestive of but not diagnostic of pregnancy failure.

Question 1.12: Regarding this image, which statement is correct?

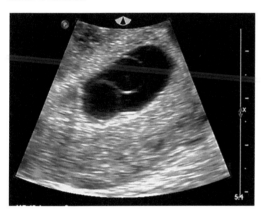

A. A multiple gestation pregnancy is not necessarily confirmed.

B. In general, a dichorionic diamniotic (DCDA) pregnancy is likely, however a monochorionic diamniotic (MCDA) pregnancy is excluded.

C. In general, a monochorionic monoamniotic (MCMA) pregnancy is excluded.

D. None of the above.

Answer:

C. Correct. The image demonstrates two yolk sacs within a gestational sac. This is consistent with a twin pregnancy. A twin pregnancy can be MCMA (2%), MCDA (30%), or DCDA (68%). In general, an MCMA twin pregnancy results from one fertilization event, typically leading to one yolk sac.

A. Incorrect. Two yolk sacs typically indicate a multiple gestation pregnancy, most commonly a twin pregnancy.

B. Incorrect. The image demonstrates two yolk sacs within a single gestational sac. The configuration is more typically seen in MCDA twins than DCDA twins. DCDA twins typically demonstrates two separate gestational sacs, each with its own yolk sac.

D. Incorrect. In general, a MCMA pregnancy is excluded since two yolk sacs are present.

Question 1.13: What structure is indicated by the *arrow*?

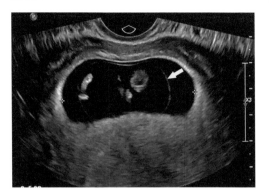

A.   Amnion.
B.   Chorion.
C.   Yolk sac.
D.   Gestational sac.

Answer:
A. Correct. Amnion. The *arrow* indicates the amniotic membrane.

B. Incorrect. The chorion is not indicated by the *arrow*.

C. Incorrect. The yolk sac is not indicated by the *arrow*.

D. Incorrect. The gestational sac is not indicated by the *arrow*.

Question 1.14: In a normal pregnancy, the amnion is usually no longer visible by the?
A.   10th week of gestation.
B.   14th week of gestation.
C.   18th week of gestation.
D.   22th week of gestation.

Answer:
B. Correct. The amnion usually fuses with the chorion by the 14th week after which it is no longer visible as a separate membrane. If seen as a separate membrane later than usual, chorioamniotic separation should be suspected, which could be a harbinger of complications.

A, C, D—Incorrect. The amnion is usually no longer visible by the 14th week.

Question 1.15: This 26-year-old female presents with a positive beta HCG and vaginal bleeding. Which statement is correct?

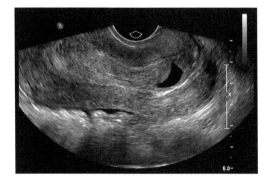

A.   An inevitable abortion in underway.
B.   Ectopic pregnancy is ruled out.
C.   Molar pregnancy is reliably excluded.
D.   Normal IUP is present.

Answer:
A. Correct. The image demonstrates a thickened endometrium with traces of fluid. Perhaps most importantly, the internal os is open and the endocervical canal is filled with soft-tissue material. This signifies a miscarriage in progress, the course of which cannot be altered.

B. Incorrect. An ectopic pregnancy should always be considered in the setting of a positive beta HCG and the absence of an IUP.

C. Incorrect. A molar pregnancy could present with a similar picture of endometrial thickening.

D. Incorrect. A normal IUP is not visualized.

Question 1.16: This patient presents with pelvic pain and a positive beta HCG. The location of the presumed gestational sac should prompt careful evaluation of which of the following?

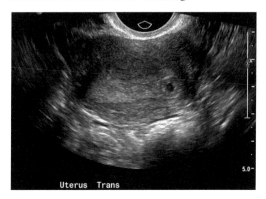

A. The size of the ovaries.
B. The myometrial mantel.
C. The endometrial thickness.
D. The beta HCG.

Answer:

B. Correct. The gestational sac is located more eccentrically than usually encountered. This brings to bear the consideration of an interstitial ectopic. This describes an ectopic pregnancy that occurs in the interstitial portion of the fallopian tube. Careful evaluation of the surrounding myometrial mantle is recommended to aid in the diagnosis since a surrounding myometrial thickness of <5 mm is suggestive of the diagnosis.

A. Incorrect. The size of the ovaries will not aid in the sonographic diagnosis of an interstitial ectopic pregnancy.

C. Incorrect. This option will not aid in the sonographic diagnosis of an interstitial ectopic pregnancy.

D. Incorrect. Serial beta HCG levels may help to predict an abnormal early pregnancy, however it would not allow the specific diagnosis of an interstitial ectopic to be made.

Question 1.17: A 27-year-old woman presents with a right adnexal pain. Regarding the presented image, which statement is correct?

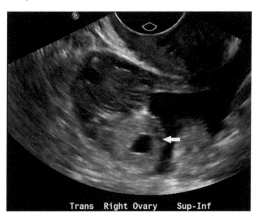

A. The *arrow* likely indicates a corpus luteal cyst.
B. If an ectopic is present, it is likely ovarian in location.
C. If the beta HCG is positive but doubles in value in 48 hours, an ectopic pregnancy is excluded.
D. None of the above.

Answer:

D. Correct. The *arrow* indicates an echogenic ring abutting, but separate from the ovary. These findings constitute the "tubal ring sign" and indicate a tubal ectopic pregnancy. Most tubal ectopic pregnancies occur within the ampullary portion of the tube.

A. Incorrect. A corpus luteal cyst is typically hypoechoic and is usually within the ovarian as opposed to abutting it.

B. Incorrect. Ectopic pregnancies very infrequently occur within the ovary. In particular, 3% of ectopic pregnancies are ovarian.

C. Incorrect. Approximately 20% of ectopic pregnancies may demonstrate doubling of beta HCG levels in 48 hours, mimicking an intrauterine pregnancy (IUP).

Question 1.18: A 41-year-old female presents with a positive pregnancy test and questionable spotting. A pelvic ultrasound is obtained. Based on the imaging below, which statement is correct?

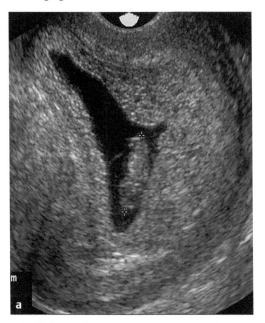

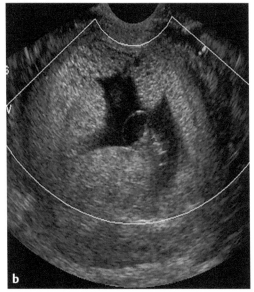

A. The appearance is within normal limits.

B. The patient probably suffers from hyperemesis.

C. A beta HCG level is likely lower than expected.

D. None of the above.

Answer:

B. Correct. The images demonstrate irregular thickening of the endometrium with numerous tiny cystic spaces. An irregular gestational sac is noted with a presumed fetal pole. The findings are suggestive of a molar pregnancy. Molar pregnancies occur in patients at extremes of age and are frequently associated with hyperemesis.

A. Incorrect. The appearance is very abnormal.

C. Incorrect. The beta HCG is often greater than expected for gestational age in molar pregnancies.

D. Incorrect. The findings are suggestive of a molar pregnancy. Molar pregnancies are frequently associated with hyperemesis.

Question 1.19: The bilateral ovaries of the patient with a molar pregnancy are shown in the below images. Each measures roughly 8 cm in maximum length. What accounts for the appearance?

A. Bilateral ovarian neoplasms.

B. Theca lutein cysts.

C. Tubo-ovarian abscesses.

D. None of the above.

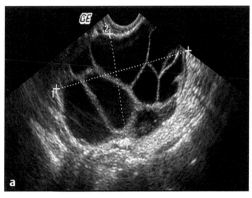

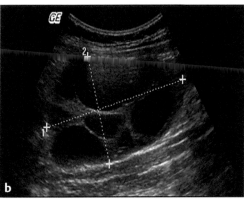

Answer:

B. Correct. Theca lutein cysts are usually noted in the enlarged ovaries of patients with molar pregnancy.

A. Incorrect. While synchronous bilateral ovarian neoplasms may occur, this option is not the most likely choice.

C. Incorrect. This option is not the most likely scenario. Tubo-ovarian abscesses usually present as complex cystic lesions with layering debris.

D. Incorrect. The findings are consistent with theca lutein cysts in the setting of a molar pregnancy.

Question 1.20: What karyotype is likely present? Refer to the images in question 1.18.

A. 23x.

B. 45xo.

C. 46 xx.

D. 69 xxy.

Answer:

D. Correct. The presence of a fetal pole within a molar pregnancy suggests a partial mole as opposed to a complete mole. A partial mole arises as a result of fertilization of one ovum by two spermatozoa. Consequently, this results in a triploid pregnancy. A complete mole is formed from the fertilization of an "empty ovum" by a haploid spermatozoon, followed by chromosomal duplication resulting in a diploid pregnancy.

A, B, C—Incorrect. A partial mole results in a triploid pregnancy.

Further Readings

Chukus A, Tirada N, Restrepo R, Reddy NI. Uncommon implantation sites of ectopic pregnancy, thinking beyond the complex adnexal mass. Radiographics 2015;35(3):946–959

Levine D, Brown DL, Andreotti RF, et al. Management of asymptomatic ovarian and other adnexal cysts imaged at US: Society of Radiologists in Ultrasound Consensus Conference Statement. Radiology 2010; 256(3):943–954

Levine D, Patel MD, Suh-Burgmann EJ, et al. Simple Adnexal Cysts: SRU Consensus Conference Update on Follow-up and Reporting. Radiology 2019 293:2, 359-371

Lin EP, Bhatt S, Dogra VS. Diagnostic clues to ectopic pregnancy. Radiographics 2008;28(6):1661–1671

Chapter 2

Second Trimester Obstetrics

Karen Tran-Harding

Questions and Answers

Refer to the following figure for questions 2.1 to 2.3.

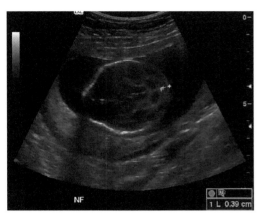

Question 2.1: What measurement is being obtained?

A. Nuchal fold.

B. Nuchal translucency.

C. Skull thickness.

D. Biparietal diameter.

Question 2.2: At what gestational age is the measurement usually obtained?

A. At 8 to 11 weeks.

B. At 11 to 14 weeks.

C. At 15 to 20 weeks.

D. At 22 to 25 weeks.

Question 2.3: Which of the following is seen on this image?

A. Lemon skull and banana sign.

B. Strawberry skull and banana sign.

C. Lemon skull and Spalding sign.

D. Strawberry skull and Spalding sign.

Answer 2.1:

A. Correct. The image demonstrates measurement of the nuchal fold. This is typically obtained in the midline, at the level of the posterior fossa. The nuchal fold is considered abnormal if it is 6 mm or greater. Increased nuchal skin thickness is a sensitive ultrasound marker for trisomy 21.

B. Incorrect. The nuchal translucency measurement is obtained more inferiorly at the level of the neck.

C, D—Incorrect. The nuchal fold is being measured.

Answer 2.2:

C. Correct. While there is some variation in the literature, the nuchal fold is obtained in the second trimester between 15 to 18–20 weeks.

A, B, D—Incorrect.

Answer 2.3:

A. Correct. The image demonstrates scalloping of the frontal bones resulting in a lemon-like shape of the skull. There is also bowing of the cerebellum with effacement of the cisterna magna. The cerebellar shape becomes reminiscent of a banana. These findings are typically encountered in Chiari II malformation and spina bifida.

B. Incorrect. Strawberry skull is seen as flattening of the occiput due to midbrain hypoplasia and flattening of the frontal bones due to frontal lobe hypoplasia. This is associated with trisomy 18.

C. Incorrect. Spalding sign is characterized by overlapping skull bones and is encountered in situations of fetal demise.

D. Incorrect. Strawberry skull and Spalding sign are not depicted in the image presented.

Question 2.4: Which of the following is true about the anomaly seen on ultrasound (US)?

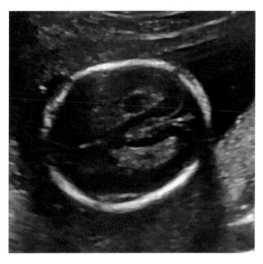

A. It is formed by infolding of the neuroepithelium and is lined by epithelium.

B. It is associated with trisomy 13.

C. Other anomalies should be sought including overlapping digits and rocker bottom deformity.

D. When this anomaly is seen, the next step is an amniocentesis for definitive diagnosis.

Answer:

C. **Correct.** The image demonstrates the classic appearance of a choroid plexus cyst, a frequent finding, though often of little clinical significance. However, there is an association with trisomy 18. For this reason, overlapping digits and rocker bottom feet should be excluded on prenatal sonographic evaluation.

A. Incorrect. Although choroid plexus cysts are formed by infolding of the neuroepithelium, it is not a true cyst and is not lined by epithelium. Rather, choroid plexus cysts are formed from spaces within the choroid plexus and are filled with clear fluid (CSF) and cellular debris.

B. Incorrect. Associations with choroid plexus cysts include trisomy 18, trisomy 21, Klinefelter's syndrome, and Aicardi syndrome. Trisomy 13 is not a known association.

D. Incorrect. Although choroid plexus cysts can be associated with chromosomal abnormalities, these can be isolated findings as well. When a choroid plexus is seen, the next best step is a triple screen.

Question 2.5: Which of the following is true given the abnormality seen on the US image? The *arrow* points to the fetal bladder.

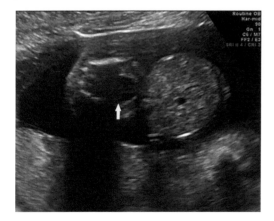

A. Other major anomalies or aneuploidies are rare.

B. This anomaly is typically located to the right of umbilical cord insertion.

C. The stomach bubble should still be visible within the abdomen.

D. The abdominal contents are only covered by a two-layer sac of amnion and peritoneum.

Answer:

D. **Correct**. The image demonstrate the classic appearance of an omphalocele, seen to the right of the image as herniated abdominal contents covered by a membrane. This membrane consists of two layers, amnion and peritoneum.

A. Incorrect. This anomaly is associated with other major anomalies or aneuploidies in over 50% of cases.

B. Incorrect. The umbilical cord inserts into the anterior part of the defect in omphaloceles.

C. Incorrect. Like gastroschisis and congenital diaphragmatic hernias, omphaloceles are associated with absence of the stomach bubble within the abdomen.

Question 2.6: What is true about the condition demonstrated within this sonographic image?

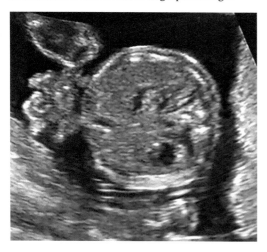

A. Associated anomalies and aneuploidies are rare.
B. It is the most common anterior abdominal wall defect of the fetus.
C. The umbilical cord inserts into the anterior part of the defect.
D. Fetal ascites is a common association.

Answer:

A. **Correct**. The image demonstrates the classic appearance of gastroschisis, with herniated abdominal contents seen to the left of the image. Associated anomalies and aneuploidies are rare.

B. Incorrect. Omphaloceles are the most common anterior abdominal wall defect of the fetus occurring in 1 in 4,000 live births. Gastroschisis occurs in 1 in 10,000 live births.

C. Incorrect. The umbilical cord inserts normally on the abdomen. The defect is usually to the right of the umbilicus. The umbilical cord inserts into the anterior part of the defect in omphaloceles.

D. Incorrect. Fetal ascites cannot occur in gastroschisis as the bowel is not covered by a membrane and floats freely in the amniotic fluid.

Question 2.7: What is true of this condition?

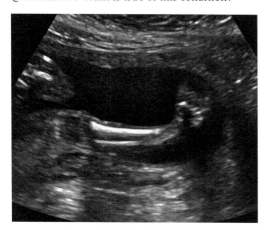

A. It is almost always unilateral.
B. It is a feared complication of early amniocentesis.
C. It does not occur in dizygotic twin gestations.
D. It is often seen in the setting of polyhydramnios.

Answer:

B. **Correct**. The image demonstrates the classic appearance of talipes equinovarus (clubfoot). Visualizing the tibia/fibula and metatarsals/phalanges on the same image is helpful in making the diagnosis on prenatal ultrasound. It is a feared complication of early amniocentesis and associated with a fourfold increase of talipes equinovarus (clubfoot) compared with chorionic villous sampling.

A. Incorrect. Clubfoot may frequently affect one or both feet.

C. Incorrect. Clubfoot may occur in any type of multifetal gestation secondary to fetal crowding.

D. Incorrect. Clubfoot is often seen in the setting of oligohydramnios, presumably caused by fixed positioning of fetal extremities due to lack of movement.

Question 2.8: Which of the following is correct regarding the imaged condition?

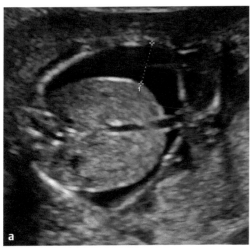

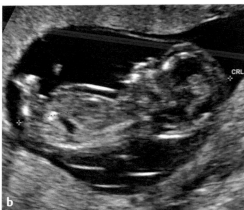

A. It is characterized by excess fluid in at least two body compartments.

B. Pericardial effusions are uncommon in this condition.

C. In the immune-mediated variety, it is most often caused by ABO blood type incompatibility.

D. Oligohydramnios is a frequent association.

Answer:

A. Correct. The images demonstrate pleural effusions and skin thickening/edema consistent with fetal hydrops. Fetal hydrops is characterized by excess fluid in at least two body compartments.

B. Incorrect. Pleural and pericardial effusions as well as ascites are typical findings.

C. Incorrect. The most common cause for the immune mediated type of fetal hydrops is rhesus (Rh) incompatibility.

D. Incorrect. Fetal hydrops is more likely to be associated with polyhydramnios.

Question 2.9: The kidneys are indicated by the *arrows*. What is true of the finding depicted in the kidney to the left of the image?

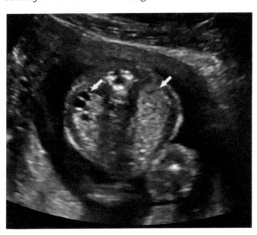

A. The renal changes occur secondary to obstruction or atresia at the level of the distal ureter.

B. The condition is characterized by multiple communicating cysts.

C. Renal cysts can be a normal finding in utero.

D. The amniotic fluid level is usually normal.

Answer:

D. Correct. The image demonstrates multiple cysts within the kidney to the left of the image. The renal parenchyma is also somewhat echogenic. The findings are consistent with multicystic dysplastic kidney (MCDK). Amniotic fluid level is usually normal in MCDK.

A. Incorrect. The renal changes of MCDK occur secondary to obstruction at the renal pelvis or the proximal ureter prior to 10 weeks.

B. Incorrect. MCDK is characterized by noncommunicating cysts that also do not communicate with the renal pelvis. Rather, ureteropelvic junction (UPJ) obstruction demonstrates fluid areas that connect, i.e., pelvocaliectasis.

C. Incorrect. MCDK occurs more often unilaterally. Bilateral MCDK can be lethal owing to oligohydramnios and pulmonary hypoplasia.

Question 2.10: Which of the following is correct about the condition depicted in the image?

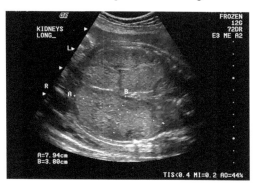

A. This condition is uniformly fatal in utero or within the first year of life.

B. This disease typically presents during the first trimester.

C. Pulmonary hypoplasia is a known complication.

D. The amniotic fluid level is usually normal.

Answer:

C. Correct. This sonographic image depicts bilaterally enlarged echogenic kidneys, filling much of the abdominal cavity. These findings are typical of autosomal recessive polycystic kidney disease (ARPKD). There is often associated oligohydramnios with thoracic hypoplasia. The narrowed thorax is noted within the right side of the sonographic image.

A. Incorrect. The juvenile form of ARPKD may result in a longer life expectancy. However, associated liver fibrosis leads to severe portal hypertension in adolescence/early adulthood.

B. Incorrect. The typical prenatal sonographic findings are usually detected during the second and third trimesters.

D. Incorrect. Oligohydramnios is associated with ARPKD.

Question 2.11: What is true about the measurement being obtained?

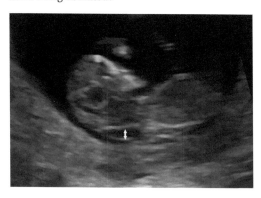

A. This measurement should be obtained between 15- and 18-week gestational age.

B. The measurement should be obtained with mild neck flexion.

C. A measurement of greater than 3 mm is abnormal.

D. An unfused amnion may lead to underestimation.

Answer:

C. Correct. The image demonstrates measurement of the nuchal translucency. This measurement is obtained at 11- to 14-week gestational age. The measurement is obtained from inner echogenic line to inner echogenic line, at the level of the neck, with the neck in neutral position. A measurement of greater than 3 mm is abnormal and signifies an increased risk for chromosomal abnormalities such as trisomy 21.

A. Incorrect. The nuchal translucency is measured between 11- and 14-week gestational age, earlier than the nuchal fold which is measured between 15 and 18–20 weeks.

B. Incorrect. The measurement of the nuchal translucency is at the level of the neck. The nuchal fold is measured at the level of the cerebellum and cisterna magna.

D. Incorrect. An unfused amnion may lead to overestimation of the nuchal translucency as the unfused amnion may be mistaken for the fetal skin line.

Question 2.12: What is true about the finding depicted in the following image?

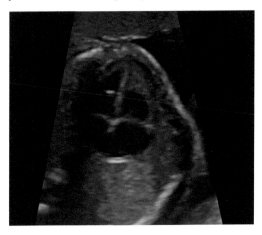

A. It represents calcification of the chordae tendineae.
B. This finding should always prompt a karyotype analysis.
C. The most common location for this finding is the right ventricle.
D. The salient finding does not usually cause shadowing.

Answer:
D. **Correct**. The sonographic image depicts an echogenic cardiac spot. These spots represent mineralization of the papillary muscle and they typically do not cast a shadow. This is likely related to their small size (usually 3 mm or less) and constant motion.

A. Incorrect. It represents mineralization of the papillary muscle.

B. Incorrect. Although the echogenic cardiac spot may be a soft marker for trisomy 21, in a low-risk population, the mildly increased risk of Down's syndrome does not require a karyotype analysis.

C. Incorrect. The most common location for this finding is the left ventricle.

Question 2.13: What is true about the finding depicted in the following image?

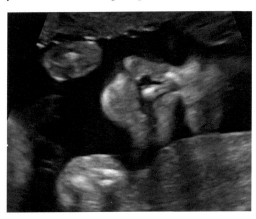

A. This anomaly affects females more often than males.
B. The finding is often bilateral when associated with holoprosencephaly.
C. Oligohydramnios is a common associated finding.
D. Fifty percent of patients with this condition will have other structural anomalies.

Answer:
D. **Correct**. The image demonstrates the classic appearance of cleft palate/lip. Approximately 50% of patients with this condition have other anomalies, such as trisomy 13 and 18. Both cleft lip and palate is found in 50%, isolated cleft lip in 20%, and isolated cleft palate in 30%.

A. Incorrect. This anomaly affects males more than females, accounting for 60 to 80% of cases.

B. Incorrect. Midline defects are often associated with holoprosencephaly.

C. Incorrect. These pregnancies are often complicated by polyhydramnios due to impaired fetal swallowing.

Question 2.14: What is true of the finding depicted in the following images?

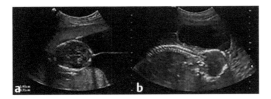

A. Turner's syndrome is the most common association.
B. About 20% of patients will have an associated chromosomal abnormality.
C. This abnormality is caused by venous dysplasia.
D. These are only seen in the posterior neck of the fetus.

Answer:

A. **Correct**. The images demonstrate a large septated cystic structure arising from the posterior neck. These findings are typical of cystic hygroma. Turner's syndrome is the most common association.

B. Incorrect. About 70% of patients will have an associated chromosomal abnormality.

C. Incorrect. This abnormality is caused by lymphatic dysplasia with subsequent leakage of the lymphatics causing localized areas of fluid collections.

D. Incorrect. Cystic hygromas can be seen elsewhere in the body including the thoracic and abdominal walls.

Question 2.15: Which is true of the finding depicted in the image below?

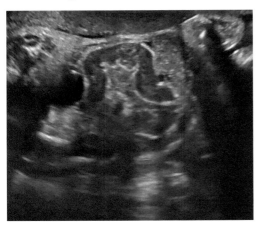

A. It is usually the earliest finding of cystic fibrosis.
B. The cause for this finding typically originates within the colon.
C. Oligohydramnios is usually present.
D. The disease that most often causes this finding is autosomal dominant.

Answer:

A. **Correct**. The image demonstrates a dilated segment of bowel. Almost all infants with dilated bowel and meconium ileus have cystic fibrosis. Dilated bowel is typically the earliest finding of cystic fibrosis.

B. Incorrect. Dilated proximal small bowel caused by thick and sticky meconium usually occurs in the terminal ileum rather than the colon.

C. Incorrect. The amniotic fluid level is usually normal or high.

D. Incorrect. Cystic fibrosis is an autosomal recessive inherited disease.

Question 2.16: Which of the following is true of the imaged condition below?

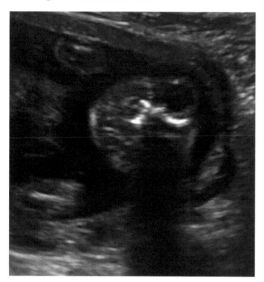

A. The diagnosis should be delayed until the early second trimester.
B. Oligohydramnios is a frequent finding.
C. The face below the orbits is usually malformed.
D. High maternal serum beta human chorionic gonadotropin level is usually present in the second trimester.

Answer:
A. **Correct**. The image demonstrates lack of supraorbital tissue consistent with anencephaly. By 12 to 14 weeks, the normal fetal head and intracranial structures can be identified. Although some of these structures can be identified via a transvaginal scan as early as 9 to 10 weeks, the definitive diagnosis of anencephaly should be made in the early second trimester.

B. Incorrect. Polyhydramnios is usually found in cases of anencephaly secondary to impaired fetal swallowing.

C. Incorrect. Although there is absence of the normal calvarium and normal brain tissue above the orbits, the face below the orbits is usually normal.

D. Incorrect. High maternal serum alpha fetoprotein level is present in the second trimester.

Question 2.17: Regarding the finding below, which statement is correct?

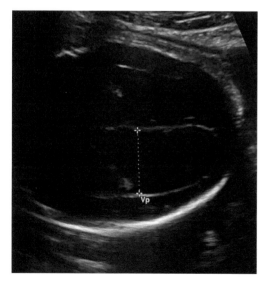

A. This finding is within normal limits.
B. The upper limit for lateral ventricular diameter is 10 mm in the second trimester and 20 mm in the third trimester.

C. The fetal prognosis is related to the cerebral cortical thickness.
D. A small amount of fluid between the choroid plexus and medial wall of the lateral ventricle is diagnostic for hydrocephalus between 18- and 20-week gestation.

Answer:
C. **Correct**. The image demonstrates severe ventriculomegaly with the classic dangling choroid plexus sign. Fetal prognosis is related to the cerebral cortical thickness.

A. Incorrect. The imaged findings are grossly abnormal.

B. Incorrect. The upper limit for lateral ventricular diameter is 10 mm throughout pregnancy.

D. Incorrect. Between 18- and 20-week gestation, a small amount of fluid between the medial wall of the lateral ventricle and the choroid plexus can be a normal finding.

Question 2.18: This sonographic image was obtained at the level of the upper abdomen. What chromosomal abnormality is most likely to be present?

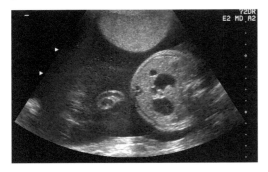

A. Trisomy 13.
B. Trisomy 18.
C. Trisomy 21.
D. Meckel–Gruber syndrome.

Answer:

C. **Correct**. The image demonstrates the classic "double bubble sign" the hallmark of duodenal atresia. Trisomy 21 is the most common chromosomal abnormality that is associated duodenal atresia.

A. Incorrect. Trisomy 13 is not typically associated with duodenal atresia.

B. Incorrect. Trisomy 18 is also not typically associated with duodenal atresia.

D. Incorrect. MeckelGruber syndrome is not typically associated with duodenal atresia.

Question 2.19: This sonographic image was obtained at the lower uterine segment in the second trimester of a 32-year-old female. What finding is demonstrated?

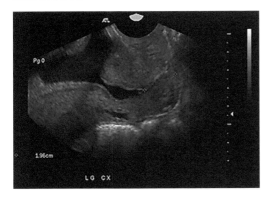

A. Cervical incompetence.
B. Placenta previa.
C. Cervical polyp.
D. Premature rupture of membranes.

Answer:

A. **Correct**. The image demonstrates a longitudinal view of the cervix showing funneling and shortening of the cervix consistent with cervical incompetence.

B. Incorrect. The placenta is not imaged.

C. Incorrect. A cervical polyp is not present.

D. Incorrect. Cervical incompetence is associated with premature rupture of membranes (PROM). The main sonographic manifestation of PROM is oligohydramnios or anhydramnios.

Question 2.20: What is the normal cervical length in pregnancy?

A. At least 2 cm.

B. At least 3 cm.

C. At least 4 cm.

D. At least 5 cm.

Answer:

B. Correct. The cervix should be at least 3 cm in length in pregnancy.

A, C, D—Incorrect.

Question 2.21: What finding is depicted in this sonogram of the lower uterine?

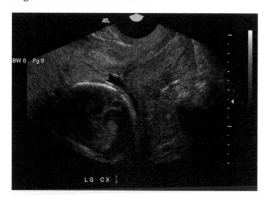

A. Marginal placenta previa.

B. Vasa previa.

C. Partial placenta previa.

D. Placental abruption.

Answer:

A. Correct. This image demonstrates the lower edge of the placenta approximating but not covering the internal os. This is consistent with marginal placenta previa.

B. Incorrect. Vasa previa is characterized by placental vessels traversing the internal os and is usually associated with a succenturiate lobe of the placenta and velamentous cord insertion. This condition may be complicated by hemorrhage from the fetal circulation and retained placenta.

C. Incorrect. In partial placenta previa the placenta covers the cervical os, albeit, incompletely.

D. Incorrect. Placental abruption is characterized by premature separation of the placenta from the uterus. This is not demonstrated in the provided image.

Further Readings

Cunningham FG, et al. Williams Obstetrics. New York, NY: McGraw-Hill Education; 2009

Doubilet PM, Benson CB. Atlas of Ultrasound in Obstetrics and Gynecology: A Multimedia Reference. Philadelphia, PA: Lippincott Williams & Wilkins; 2012

Elsayes KM, Trout AT, Friedkin AM, et al. Imaging of the placenta: a multimodality pictorial review. Radiographics 2009;29(5):1371–1391

Middleton WD, Kurtz AB, Hertzberg BS. Ultrasound: The Requisites. St. Louis, Mo: Mosby; 2004

Spalding AB. A pathognomonic sign of intra-uterine death. Surg Gynecol Obstetrics 1922;34:754

Chapter 3

Pediatrics

Edward Richer

Questions and Answers

Question 3.1: Which is true regarding the key finding in image (**a**)?

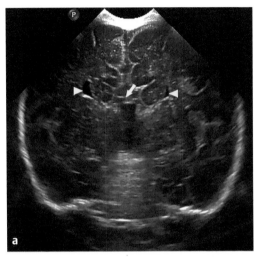

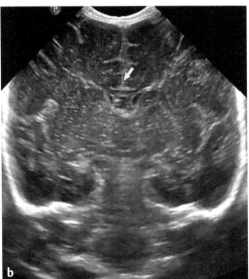

A. It is most commonly the sequela of prematurity.

B. It is commonly associated with other structural abnormalities, including Chiari I and II.

C. Frequent cause of hydrocephalus.

D. Occurs due to an abnormality of posterior to anterior development.

Answer:

B. Correct. This coronal image from a cranial ultrasound demonstrates agenesis of the corpus callosum (ACC), which is commonly associated with other structural brain anomalies, including Chiari malformations. Note the absence of the normal thin, hypoechoic corpus in image (**a**, *arrow*), compared to the normal corpus in image (**b**, *arrow*). Also note the widely spaced lateral ventricles (*arrowheads*), a finding which has been termed the "Texas Longhorn" or "Bullwinkle" sign.

A. Incorrect. ACC is a developmental disorder, not related to prematurity.

C. Incorrect. ACC in and of itself does not cause hydrocephalus.

D. Incorrect. The corpus callosum develops in an anterior to posterior direction.

Question 3.2: What is the most reliable sonographic feature of this diagnosis?

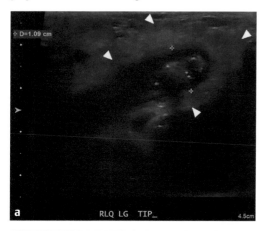

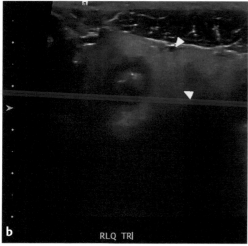

A. Diameter greater than 6 mm.
B. Free fluid in the right lower quadrant.
C. Abnormal hyperemia.
D. Increased echotexture of adjacent fat.

Answer:

D. Correct. Longitudinal and transverse images demonstrate a dilated appendix measuring 1.1 cm with loss of normal wall echotexture, shadowing appendicolith, and increased echotexture of the periappendiceal fat (*arrowheads*). Multiple sonographic features are considered in the diagnosis of acute appendicitis, including diameter, presence of appendicolith, hyperemia, echogenic fat, free fluid, and presence of abscess; however, echogenic fat has been shown to have the strongest association with acute appendicitis, odds ratio 63–69.

A. Incorrect. There is overlap between abnormal and normal cases, with some normal appendices measuring over 6 mm and some abnormal cases less than 6 mm. Odds ratio 13–15.

B. Incorrect. Free fluid is nonspecific and has an odds ratio of 1.7 for appendicitis.

C. Incorrect. Abnormal hyperemia has a greater odds ratio for appendicitis than diameter (OR = 21), but not as great as echogenic fat.

Question 3.3: Which is true regarding this condition?

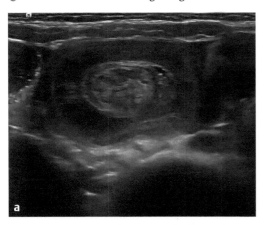

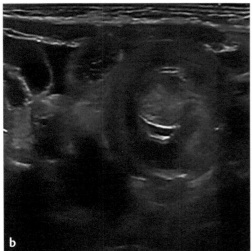

A. The patient may have presented with crampy abdominal pain and bloody stools.

B. The patient is typically taken immediately to surgery.

C. No treatment is required as this condition is usually transient and resolves spontaneously.

D. The patient is likely in the age range of 5 to 7 years.

Answer:

A. Correct. Transverse images demonstrate the typical targetoid appearance of an ileocolic intussusception. Patient symptoms are variable, but may include fussiness, lethargy, intermittent crampy or colicky abdominal pain, and occasionally, bloody stools. Radiographs are normal in up to 50% of cases, and for this reason, ultrasound is the first-line test for intussusception. Classic findings include the "target" sign on transverse images and the "pseudokidney" sign on longitudinal images.

B. Incorrect. Therapeutic enema in radiology is typically attempted prior to surgical intervention.

C. Incorrect. Ileocolic intussusception requires definitive treatment with enema or surgery to prevent bowel ischemia. Enteroenteric intussusceptions are smaller and are generally transient in nature.

D. Incorrect. The typical age range for idiopathic ileocolic intussusception is 3 months to 3 years. An older patient with intussusception raises the possibility of a pathologic lead point.

Question 3.4: Technical factors which could obscure the area of interest and prevent accurate diagnosis of this condition include all but which of the following options?

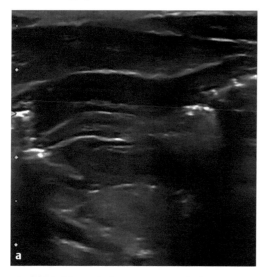

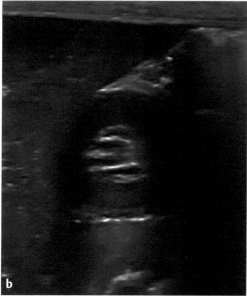

A. Overdistention of the stomach, displacing the pylorus posteriorly.

B. Patient in right anterior oblique (RAO) position, causing shadowing gas to collect in the gastric antrum and pylorus.

C. Imaging the patient while actively feeding from a bottle.

D. Imaging for a short duration, 1 to 2 minutes.

Answer:

C. **Correct**. Longitudinal and transverse images through the pylorus show an abnormally thick-walled and elongated pylorus consistent with hypertrophic pyloric stenosis (HPS). Criteria for HPS include a muscle wall thickness ≥3 mm and a channel length ≥17 mm. Having the patient drink formula, breast milk, or sugar water is often utilized during ultrasound to partially distend the stomach and visualize gastric contents emptying through the pylorus.

A. Incorrect. An overdistended stomach causes the pylorus to be displaced posteriorly/deeper into the abdomen, which can then limit visualization.

B. Incorrect. RAO position causes gas to collect in the distal stomach and may obscure visualization. If this occurs, rolling the patient into left anterior oblique position may displace gas away from the pylorus.

D. Incorrect. Imaging for a short duration may inaccurately diagnose transient pyloric thickening from pylorospasm as true HPS.

Question 3.5: Which finding in this case is most suggestive of the correct diagnosis?

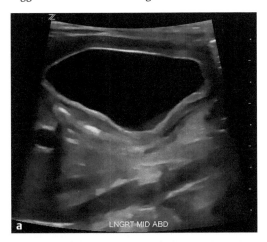

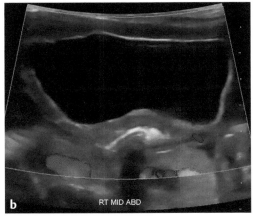

A. Alternating echogenic and hypoechoic layers.

B. Absence of vascular flow.

C. Location within the abdomen.

D. Size of the lesion.

Answer:

A. Correct. A cystic structure is demonstrated in the right mid abdomen with a wall consisting of alternating echogenic and hypoechoic layers, also known as "gut signature." The inner echogenic layer represents mucosa, while the hypoechoic layer represents the muscularis layer in this gastrointestinal duplication cyst. Occasionally, the outer echogenic serosal layer can also be seen. This alternating wall echotexture strongly suggests the diagnosis of gastrointestinal duplication cyst over other abdominal cysts, such as choledochal or ovarian cysts, or meconium pseudocysts.

B. Incorrect. Absence of vascular flow does not differentiate between pediatric abdominal cysts.

C. Incorrect. Gastrointestinal duplication cysts can occur anywhere in the abdomen, and ovaries/ovarian cysts can be large or located high in the abdomen in newborn females.

D. Incorrect. The size of the lesion does not reliably differentiate pediatric abdominal cysts.

Question 3.6: Which other organ is most likely to be affected in this newborn infant?

A. Pancreas.
B. Adrenals.
C. Spleen.
D. Liver.

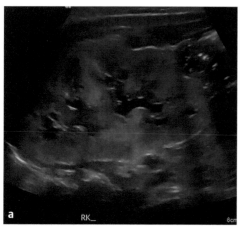

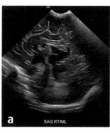

Answer:

D. Correct. Sagittal images of both kidneys in this newborn infant demonstrate bilateral enlarged, echogenic kidneys with numerous small cysts consistent with autosomal recessive polycystic kidney disease (ARPKD). Infants with ARPKD classically present with Potter sequence sequelae and pulmonary hypoplasia due oligohydramnios in utero. The liver is also affected in ARPKD, typically inversely proportional to the severity of renal involvement. Liver fibrosis and cysts are the most commonly encountered findings.

A, B, C—Incorrect. The mentioned organs are not typically involved in ARPKD.

Question 3.7: Based on the ultrasound images, which of the following option would you recommend?

A. Abdominal ultrasound to evaluate for liver hemangiomas.
B. Chest computed tomography (CT) to evaluate for arteriovenous malformations (Osler–Weber–Rendu syndrome).
C. Chest radiograph to evaluate for heart failure.
D. Positron emission tomography (PET)-CT to evaluate for associated metastases.

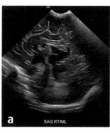

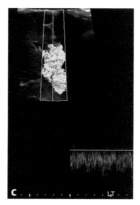

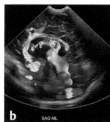

Answer:

C. Correct. Sagittal images from a cranial ultrasound show an abnormal, prominent vascular structure with venous blood flow in the posterior aspect of the brain in this neonate. The location and ultrasound appearance are characteristic for vein of Galen (VOG) malformation, or median prosencephalic arteriovenous fistula. This is a rare malformation, but is classically associated with high output heart failure due to arteriovenous shunting, with up to 80% of cardiac output shunting through the lesion. A chest radiograph would help to assess for heart failure.

A, B, D—Incorrect. VOG malformation is not associated with liver hemangiomas.

Question 3.8: The Doppler examination in this infant with elevated liver enzymes is best described as which of the following?

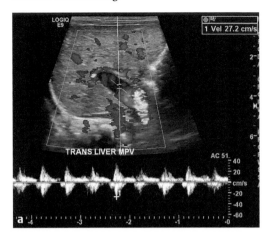

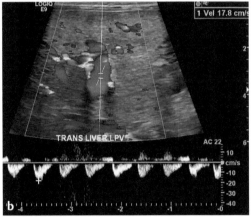

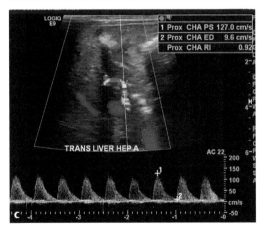

A. Normal hepatic artery and portal venous flow and waveforms.

B. Normal hepatic artery flow and waveforms, reversed flow, and arterialized waveform in portal vein.

C. Parvus tardus waveform in hepatic artery indicative of arterial stenosis, normal portal vein flow.

D. Normal hepatic artery flow, abnormal portal vein Doppler is artifactual due to incorrect Doppler angle settings.

Answer:

B. Correct. Doppler imaging of the liver shows abnormal reversal of blood flow in the main and left portal vein with arterialized waveforms. The hepatic artery waveforms and direction of flow are normal. Portal vein flow should be toward the transducer (hepatopetal), except in the posterior division of the right portal vein in which flow is away from the transducer due to the anatomy of the portal vein. Reversal of portal vein flow can be seen in severe portal hypertension, or in arteriovenous shunting, which was the diagnosis in this case.

A. Incorrect. The portal vein flow and waveforms are abnormal.

C. Incorrect. The arterial waveform is normal and does not show parvus tardus morphology.

D. Incorrect. The Doppler angle appears appropriately selected and would not produce an arterialized portal vein waveform even if incorrectly selected.

Question 3.9 In a patient with this condition, constant urinary incontinence or dribbling may be an indication of what finding? What imaging study could further evaluate for that finding?

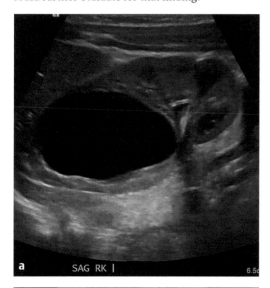

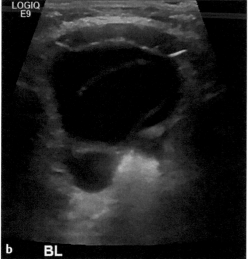

A. Ectopic ureter inserting on the urethra or vagina; magnetic resonance urography could be performed.

B. Detrusor muscle instability; urodynamic study could be performed.

C. Severe hydronephrosis; MAG3 exam with Lasix could be performed.

D. Neurogenic bladder; fluoroscopy cystogram could be performed.

Answer:

A. Correct. The images demonstrate a renal duplication, with asymmetric collecting system dilatation in the upper pole of the right kidney, and a right-sided ureterocele within the bladder. In renal duplications, the upper moiety ureter tends to insert inferomedially (Weigert-Meyer rule), and in some cases it may insert ectopically on structures other than the bladder, such as vagina, urethra, or seminal vesicles. Insertion on a structure without a sphincter mechanism, such as the vagina, can produce constant urinary dribbling and incontinence. Magnetic resonance (MR) urography would be the best choice for further imaging in children, as the ectopic insertion would be well demonstrated without exposing the patient to radiation.

B. Incorrect. Detrusor muscle instability could produce intermittent incontinence, but not constant wetness as in this patient.

C. Incorrect. Hydronephrosis would not produce incontinence.

D. Incorrect. Neurogenic bladder could produce intermittent incontinence, but not constant wetness as in this patient.

Question 3.10 Newborn infant undergoing ultrasound for hydronephrosis detected on prenatal ultrasound. A left suprarenal space lesion was incidentally discovered when imaging the left kidney, shown in the images below. What are your recommendations for management?

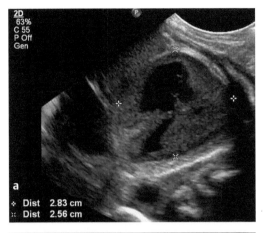

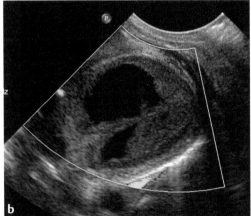

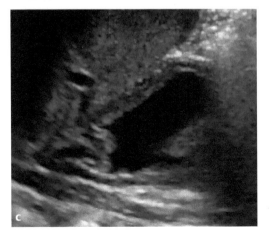

A. Urgent referral to pediatric surgeon for resection.

B. Abdominal MRI for further characterization.

C. Short-term follow-up ultrasound.

D. Image-guided biopsy by interventional radiology.

Answer:

C. Correct. The images show a complex solid and cystic left suprarenal mass. In a newborn infant, the main differential diagnosis is adrenal hemorrhage and neonatal neuroblastoma. The lack of blood flow on Doppler imaging is more suggestive of hemorrhage. Since neonatal neuroblastoma has a relatively good prognosis, an adrenal mass in a newborn can be safely followed by short-term ultrasound to evaluate for changes. On follow-up imaging, there was a decrease in overall size and solid components of the lesion, as expected for hemorrhage. Neuroblastoma would be expected to remain stable in size if not enlarge.

A. Incorrect. Adrenal hemorrhage does not require surgical resection. Neonatal neuroblastoma is not urgently resected either.

B. Incorrect. Ultrasound would be logistically easier and more cost effective to follow this lesion than MRI.

D. Incorrect. The findings are suggestive of hemorrhage and biopsy is not indicated.

Question 3.11: An otherwise healthy 9-year-old female undergoing renal ultrasound for urinary tract infections. Possible explanations for these findings include all but which of the following options?

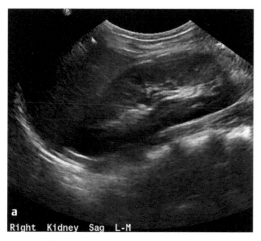

Right Kidney Sag L-M

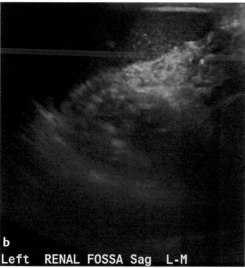

Left RENAL FOSSA Sag L-M

A. Severe renal scarring and atrophy due to multiple infections ("the wasted kidney").

B. Pelvic kidney.

C. Crossed fused ectopia.

D. Involuted multicystic dysplastic kidney (MCDK).

Answer:

A. Correct. Images of both renal fossae show a normal right kidney, with an empty left renal fossa other than spleen and bowel gas. No normal left renal tissue is seen. The sonographer should be directed to scan the pelvis to evaluate for pelvic kidney and closely examine the lower pole of the right kidney to look for crossed fused ectopia. If renal ectopia is not found, other explanations of an empty renal fossa include renal agenesis, involuted MCDK, or prior nephrectomy. Multiple urinary tract infections can produce renal scarring and atrophy, but not typically to the point that the kidney is no longer visualized.

B, C, D—Incorrect. This condition can produce an empty renal fossa.

Question 3.12: Three-month-old male with hydronephrosis on prenatal ultrasound, undergoing first postnatal ultrasound. Based on the provided images, what would be the most appropriate next step in management to confirm the diagnosis?

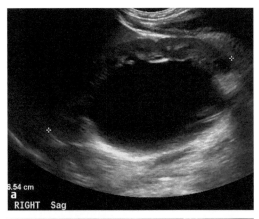

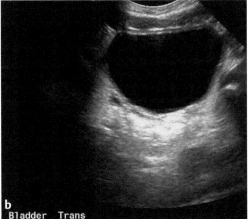

A. Voiding cystourethrogram for posterior urethral valves (PUV).

B. Abdominal and pelvic CT for distal ureteral stone.

C. Referral to urology for urgent ureteral stent placement.

D. MAG3 scan for ureteropelvic junction obstruction (UPJO).

Answer:

D. Correct. The first image shows a markedly dilated right renal pelvis with slight calyceal dilation. The second image shows a normal smooth walled urinary bladder with no distal ureteral dilation. The combination of findings is consistent with UPJO. The cause of UPJO in children is not entirely clear, but is thought to most commonly be due to abnormal smooth muscle at the UPJ preventing normal relaxation. Another cause in some cases is due to a blood vessel crossing and compressing the UPJ. The contralateral kidney should be evaluated for associated anomalies, including duplication and MCDK. MAG3 with Lasix is the most appropriate next step in management, as the exam will confirm delayed drainage through the obstructed system.

A. Incorrect. The smooth bladder wall and lack of ureteral dilation argue against posterior urethral valves.

B. Incorrect. Obstructing renal stones are uncommon in infants and the pelvic morphology is suggestive of UPJO.

C. Incorrect. Typical surgery for UPJO is pyeloplasty rather than ureteral stent placement.

Question 3.13: Ten-year-old female with mildly elevated TSH, sent for thyroid ultrasound to exclude nodule or goiter. What next step could best confirm the diagnosis?

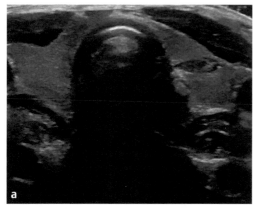

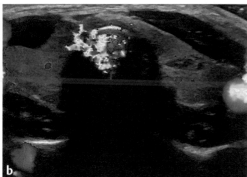

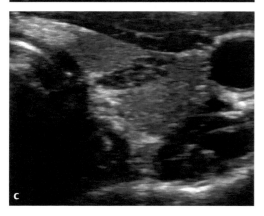

A. This is a benign colloid cyst and no further workup is needed.

B. Comparison ultrasound imaging of another organ.

C. Percutaneous ultrasound-guided fine needle aspiration (FNA), as the nodule is concerning for papillary thyroid cancer.

D. Neck CT with contrast for surgical planning.

Answer:

B. Correct. The initial images show an ovoid nodule in the left thyroid lobe with thin internal septations and small echogenic foci. There is no internal vascular flow, calcification, or capsule. The nodule does not have more typical spongiform appearance of a colloid nodule and there is no comet-tail artifact. Imaging of the thymus confirmed that the nodule had identical echotexture. The nodule was consistent with ectopic intrathyroidal thymic tissue. During gestation, the thymus arises from the third and fourth pharyngeal pouches and migrates caudally to its normal intrathoracic position. Ectopic thymic rests can occur anywhere along the path of descent.

A. Incorrect. The sonographic characteristics of the nodule are not suggestive of colloid cyst.

C. Incorrect. The imaging features are not suggestive of cancer, and FNA does not need to be performed to confirm ectopic thymic tissue given the appearance is identical to the thymus.

D. Incorrect. CT would not characterize this lesion better than ultrasound.

Question 3.14: Fourteen-year-old male, renal ultrasound with Doppler to evaluate hypertension refractory to two medications. A renal angiogram is also shown. Which of the following is true regarding this condition?

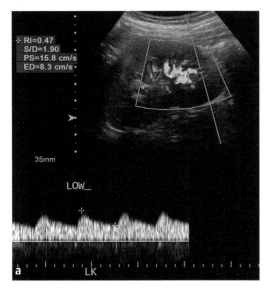

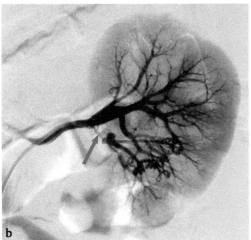

A. Grayscale images tend to show an enlarged, echogenic kidney.
B. A renal artery to aortic velocity ratio (RAR) over 1 is highly suggestive of the diagnosis.
C. A negative ultrasound excludes the diagnosis.
D. A potential cause in children is neurofibromatosis.

Answer:

D. Correct. Multiple Doppler images of the left kidney showed normal waveforms and resistive indices within arcuate arteries in the upper and mid kidney. The waveform in the lower pole showed a prolonged systolic upstroke and a low resistive index, suggesting a proximal stenotic lesion. The patient underwent renal angiography which confirmed a segmental arterial stenosis to the lower pole (*arrow*) in image **b**. In children, fibromuscular dysplasia is the cause of renal artery stenosis in up to 70% of patients, with other etiologies including neurofibromatosis, tuberous sclerosis, and inflammatory arteritides.

A. Incorrect. Grayscale images in renal artery stenosis show an atrophic, echogenic kidney.

B. Incorrect. The RAR is considered to be abnormal at 3.5 or greater.

C. Incorrect. A normal renal ultrasound does not exclude renal artery stenosis, and further imaging with CT or MR angiography, or conventional angiography, should be performed when clinical suspicion is high.

Question 3.15: Two-month-old infant, born at 26 weeks gestation, undergoing evaluation for poor feeding and generalized hypotonia. The findings on these images are secondary to which of the following?

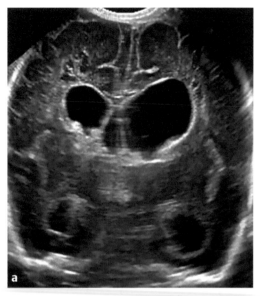

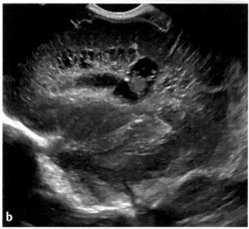

A. Prior parenchymal hemorrhage with subsequent necrosis.

B. In utero toxoplasmosis, other (syphilis, varicella-zoster, parvovirus B19), rubella, cytomegalovirus (CMV), and herpes (TORCH) infection.

C. Prior hypoxic/ischemic insult.

D. Postnatal cryptococcal infection (gelatinous pseudocysts).

Answer:

C. Correct. Coronal and sagittal images of the brain show multiple small cystic spaces in the periventricular white matter bilaterally, but more so on the right. Mild ventriculomegaly is present. This appearance, in conjunction with patient's history of prematurity, is consistent with cystic periventricular leukomalacia (PVL). PVL results from an ischemic insult to a watershed zone, which in premature infants is in the periventricular white matter. Sonographic findings of PVL include abnormal increased echotexture of the white matter or frank cystic change, as in this case. PVL can be focal or diffuse, symmetric right to left, or asymmetric. Findings typically appear on ultrasounds days to weeks after the insult.

A. Incorrect. Prior parenchymal hemorrhage with necrosis would tend to form a single cystic cavity, rather than the multiple small cysts as in this case.

B. Incorrect. TORCH infections may produce periventricular and parenchymal calcifications rather than cysts.

D. Incorrect. Gelatinous pseudocysts tend to form in the basal ganglia and are seen in immunosuppressed patients.

Question 3.16: Six-month-old infant undergoing abdominal ultrasound for mildly elevated liver enzymes. How could the sonographer be directed to increase the confidence in the most likely diagnosis?

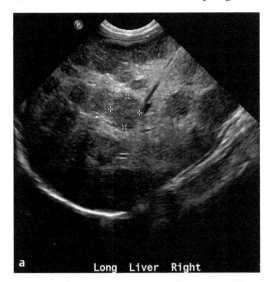

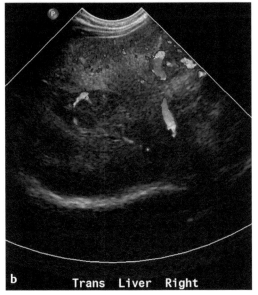

A. Increase the pulse repetition frequency to eliminate Doppler aliasing.

B. Scan the adrenal glands to evaluate for mass.

C. Scan the spleen to evaluate for additional lesions.

D. Decrease the focal zone to improve near field resolution.

Answer:

B. Correct. The images show multiple hypoechoic lesions throughout the liver with internal vascular flow. The main differential for these lesions in an infant is multiple infantile hepatic hemangiomas and metastatic disease, most commonly from neuroblastoma. The sonographer could be directed to scan the adrenal glands to evaluate for mass; if none is seen, this increases the confidence in the diagnosis of hemangiomas. Infantile hepatic hemangiomas can be single or multiple, and are most commonly treated with watchful waiting as they spontaneously involute. Symptomatic hemangiomas can result in high output heart failure or consumptive coagulopathy (Kasabach–Merritt syndrome), and may be treated with medications, embolization, or liver transplantation in extreme cases.

A. Incorrect. No significant aliasing is seen on the Doppler image, and the focal zone appears appropriate on this image.

C. Incorrect. Additional hypoechoic splenic lesions might be seen if abscesses are suspected in an immunosuppressed patient, however abscesses should not have internal blood flow.

D. Incorrect. No significant aliasing is seen on the Doppler image, and the focal zone appears appropriate on this image.

Question 3.17: Two different operators made the same mistake in two different pyloric ultrasounds. What was it?

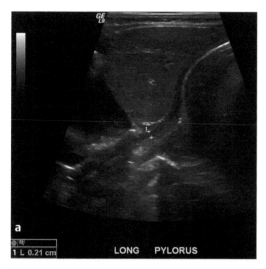

a

1 L 0.21 cm   LONG   PYLORUS

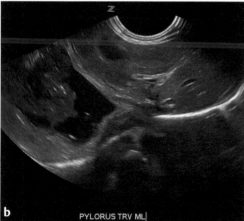

b

PYLORUS TRV ML|

A. Wrong focal zone setting.
B. Wrong measurement of pyloric wall thickness.
C. Imaging with the stomach too full.
D. Wrong body part.

Answer:

D. Correct. Both operators mistakenly imaged the gastroesophageal junction thinking it was the pylorus. The appearance can be quite similar to the pylorus, since there are layers of echogenic mucosa and hypoechoic muscularis which are closely apposed to each other. The key to avoiding this mistake is to identify landmarks which are not normally present when the pylorus is correctly imaged, such as the heart and the diaphragm.

A, B, C—Incorrect. These options were not the specific mistake.

Question 3.18: Six-week-old male with palpable right neck mass. Based on the provided images, what is the most appropriate neck step in management?

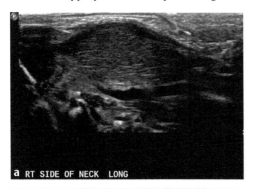

a RT SIDE OF NECK LONG

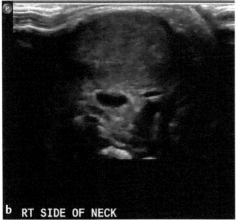

b RT SIDE OF NECK

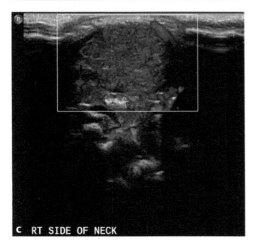

c RT SIDE OF NECK

A. Image the contralateral neck for comparison.
B. CT neck with contrast to evaluate for metastatic adenopathy and for surgical planning.
C. MRI neck to avoid radiation in this young infant.
D. The mass should be biopsied by FNA prior to any additional imaging.

Answer:

A. Correct. Longitudinal and transverse images of the right neck show an ovoid, hypervascular mass. Careful inspection of the images reveals that the mass is actually fusiform enlargement of the sternocleidomastoid (SCM) muscle, as muscle fibers can be seen, especially on the longitudinal image. This is consistent with fibromatosis colli, a benign and typically self-limited proliferation of fibrous tissue within the SCM that is the most common cause of neonatal torticollis. The key to recognizing fibromatosis colli are to appreciate that the muscle itself is enlarged, and comparison imaging of the contralateral SCM showing normal muscle can help to confirm the diagnosis.

B. Incorrect. Additional imaging with CT is not indicated when the sonographic features are consistent with fibromatosis colli. If the mass did not have the typical appearance or was more aggressive, cross-sectional imaging could be indicated.

C. Incorrect. Additional imaging with MRI is not indicated when the sonographic features are consistent with fibromatosis colli. If the mass did not have the typical appearance or was more aggressive, cross-sectional imaging could be indicated.

D. Incorrect. An invasive procedure such as biopsy is certainly not indicated in this benign condition.

Question 3.19: Seven-day-old late preterm infant in NICU for mild respiratory distress, noted to have hematuria and decreasing platelet counts. In neonates, which of the following is not a potential cause of this condition?

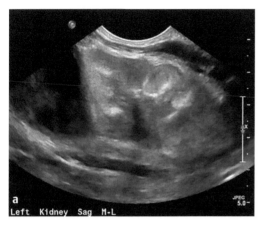

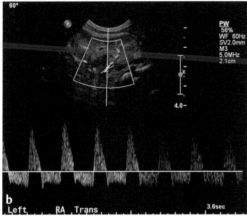

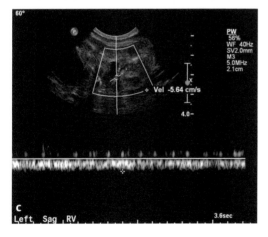

A. Dehydration.
B. Sepsis/infection.
C. Maternal diabetes.
D. Vesicoureteral reflux.

Answer:

D. Correct. The images show an echogenic left kidney with poor corticomedullary differentiation and linear echogenic structures. The Doppler images show reversal of diastolic blood flow in the main renal artery and a dampened, monophasic waveform in the main renal vein. The imaging findings and clinical symptoms are consistent with renal vein thrombosis (RVT), albeit, non-occlusive since some dampened flow is detected with the renal vein. Causes of RVT in neonates include dehydration or hypotension from any source, including sepsis and congenital heart disease, and maternal diabetes, among others. Central lines such as peripherally inserted central catheters within the inferior vena cava can also serve as a nidus for thrombosis. Vesicoureteral reflux is not a cause of RVT.

A, B, C—Incorrect. These are known causes of RVT.

Question 3.20: Three-week-old male undergoing workup for hydronephrosis on prenatal ultrasound. What is the most appropriate next step?

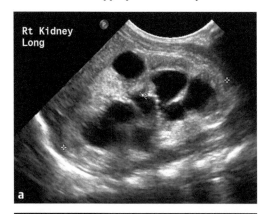

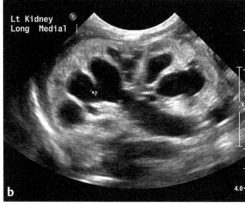

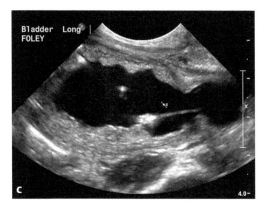

A. MAG3 scan with Lasix.
B. Voiding cystourethrography (VCUG).
C. MR urography.
D. Percutaneous nephrostomy.

Answer:

B. Correct. The images show bilateral hydronephrosis, and a small volume, thick walled and irregular bladder. In a male, these findings are highly suggestive of posterior urethral valves (PUV). In fact, the finding of bilateral hydronephrosis in a male patient should prompt workup for valves. The image of the bladder shows the classic "keyhole" sign made by the bladder, bladder neck, and dilated posterior urethra. VCUG is the most appropriate next step to confirm the diagnosis, and will demonstrate a dilated posterior urethra with abrupt caliber change at the level of the valves to a small caliber anterior urethra.

A. Incorrect. MAG3 scans with Lasix are more suitable for evaluating unilateral obstructions such as ureteropelvic or ureterovesicular junction obstructions.

C. Incorrect. Quicker, easier, and less expensive test for PUV is VCUG.

D. Incorrect. Percutaneous nephrostomy will do nothing to alleviate the urethral obstruction.

Further Readings

Applegate KE. Intussusception in children: evidence-based diagnosis and treatment. Pediatr Radiol 2009; 39(Suppl 2):S140–S143

Ablin DS, Jain K, Howell L, West DC. Ultrasound and MR imaging of fibromatosis colli (sternomastoid tumor of infancy). Pediatr Radiol 1998;28(4):230–233

Barkovich AJ, Norman D. Anomalies of the corpus callosum: correlation with further anomalies of the brain. AJR Am J Roentgenol 1988;151(1):171–179

Berrocal T, López-Pereira P, Arjonilla A, Gutiérrez J. Anomalies of the distal ureter, bladder, and urethra in children: embryologic, radiologic, and pathologic features. Radiographics 2002;22(5):1139–1164

Castelli PK, Dillman JR, Kershaw DB, Khalatbari S, Stanley JC, Smith EA. Renal sonography with Doppler for detecting suspected pediatric renin-mediated hypertension—is it adequate? Pediatr Radiol 2014;44(1):42–49

Heij HA, Taets van Amerongen AH, Ekkelkamp S, Vos A. Diagnosis and management of neonatal adrenal haemorrhage. Pediatr Radiol 1989;19(6-7):391–394

Hernanz-Schulman M. Infantile hypertrophic pyloric stenosis. Radiology 2003;227(2):319–331

Hibbert J, Howlett DC, Greenwood KL, MacDonald LM, Saunders AJ. The ultrasound appearances of neonatal renal vein thrombosis. Br J Radiol 1997;70(839):1191–1194

Jones BV, Ball WS, Tomsick TA, Millard J, Crone KR. Vein of Galen aneurysmal malformation: diagnosis and treatment of 13 children with extended clinical follow-up. AJNR Am J Neuroradiol 2002;23(10):1717–1724

Kassarjian A, Zurakowski D, Dubois J, Paltiel HJ, Fishman SJ, Burrows PE. Infantile hepatic hemangiomas: clinical and imaging findings and their correlation with therapy. AJR Am J Roentgenol 2004; 182(3):785–795

Kim HG, Kim MJ, Lee MJ. Sonographic appearance of intrathyroid ectopic thymus in children. J Clin Ultrasound 2012;40(5):266–271

Lonergan GJ, Rice RR, Suarez ES. Autosomal recessive polycystic kidney disease: radiologic-pathologic correlation. Radiographics 2000;20(3):837–855

McNaughton DA, Abu-Yousef MM. Doppler US of the liver made simple. Radiographics 2011;31(1):161–188

Mercado-Deane MG, Beeson JE, John SD. US of renal insufficiency in neonates. Radiographics 2002;22(6): 1429–1438

Puligandla PS, Nguyen LT, St-Vil D, et al. Gastrointestinal duplications. J Pediatr Surg 2003;38(5): 740–744

Seigel M. Pediatric Sonography. 4th ed. Philadelphia, PA: Lippincott Williams & Wilkins; 2010

Shapiro E, Goldfarb DA, Ritchey ML. The congenital and acquired solitary kidney. Rev Urol 2003;5(1):2–8

Trout AT, Sanchez R, Ladino-Torres MF. Reevaluating the sonographic criteria for acute appendicitis in children: a review of the literature and a retrospective analysis of 246 cases. Acad Radiol 2012;19(11): 1382–1394

Chapter 4

Renal

Adrian Dawkins

4 Questions and Answers

Question 4.1: Longitudinal sonogram of the right kidney obtained in a 35-year-old male with acute renal failure. What anatomic structure is indicated by the *arrow*?

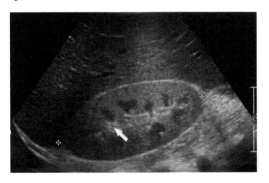

A. Renal cortex.
B. Renal medulla.
C. Position of arcuate arteries.
D. Renal sinus.

Answer:

D. Correct. The area indicated is the echogenic renal sinus fat that surrounds the renal collecting system and vessels.

A. Incorrect. The renal cortex is the outermost layer of the kidney.

B. Incorrect. The medullary pyramids are found deep to the outer renal cortex and form part of the renal parenchyma. They are typically hypo- to isoechoic with respect to the outer cortex.

C. Incorrect. The arcuate arteries are positioned more peripherally within the renal parenchyma and run along the border of the cortex and medullary pyramids.

Question 4.2: Which statement is correct?
A. In the adult population, the kidneys are usually more echogenic than the normal liver.
B. When the liver extends below the inferior pole of the right kidney, hepatomegaly is present.
C. The kidneys move inferiorly with inspiration.
D. In neonates, the renal cortex is typically hypoechoic with respect to the liver.

Answer:
C. Correct. Both kidneys move inferiorly during inspiration. This maneuver may be used to improve visualization of the kidneys as well as to facilitate image-guided renal biopsies.

A. Incorrect. In the adult patient, the normal kidney is usually hypoechoic with respect to the liver. The renal cortex in this case demonstrates abnormally increased echogenicity secondary to acute tubular necrosis.

B. Incorrect. While the liver may extend below the right kidney in hepatomegaly, this may also be a normal variant, Riedel's lobe. Other coexisting findings such as rounding of the inferior liver edge or actual volume measurements using 3D ultrasound are better predictors of hepatomegaly.

D. Incorrect. In neonates, the renal cortex is typically hyperechoic with respect to the liver.

Question 4.3: A longitudinal sonographic view of the left kidney is obtained in a 45-year-old male with suspected left renal colic. Which statement is correct?

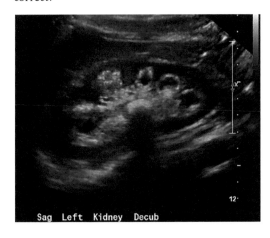

Sag Left Kidney Decub

A. Ultrasound is the first test of choice in the diagnosis of this condition, in this patient population.

B. The composition of the calculus may be inferred from the imaging appearances.

C. Calcium oxalate calculi are the most common type.

D. Pure uric acid stones are not visible on ultrasound.

Answer:

C. Correct. Renal calculi develop from a variety of reasons and therefore tend to vary in chemical composition. However, roughly 80% of renal calculi are calcium based with calcium oxalate stone accounting for roughly 60% of all calculi.

A. Incorrect. Noncontrast computed tomography (CT) is the investigation of choice in adults and nonpregnant females in the setting of suspected renal colic.

B. Incorrect. The composition of renal calculi cannot be directly inferred from ultrasound appearances alone since stones of differing composition may have similar sonographic appearances.

D. Incorrect. Uric acid stones may not be visible on plain radiographs. However, these stones are dense enough to be discerned sonographically.

Question 4.4: Which statement is correct regarding the stone size?

A. Spatial compounding is more accurate than harmonic imaging at estimating stone size.

B. Posterior acoustic shadow width is touted as being a more accurate estimate of true stone size with increasing kidney depth.

C. The smaller the stone, the more accurate the sonographic measurement.

D. Ultrasound tends to underestimate the size of stones.

Answer:

B. Correct. With increasing depth, ultrasound tends to overestimate the size of calculi, since the ultrasound beam diverges beyond the focal zone. However, the posterior acoustic shadow cast by the stone is less affected by this phenomenon.

A. Incorrect. Spatial compounding seeks to improve image uniformity by obtaining data from multiple scan angles. This results in reduction of conspicuity of stone and shadow boundaries, leading to errors in size measurements. Harmonic imaging augments imaging by adding data obtained from higher frequencies. This improves lateral resolution and hence results in a more accurate estimate of actual stone size. However, this comes at the expense of signal to noise and depth penetration.

C. Incorrect. The smaller the stone, the greater the error in measurement especially if the stone is <5 mm.

D. Incorrect. Ultrasound tends to overestimate the size of stones.

Question 4.5: A longitudinal view of a transplanted kidney is presented with color and spectral Doppler analysis. What is the diagnosis?

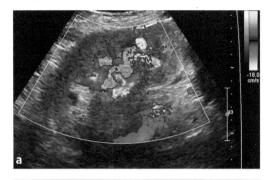

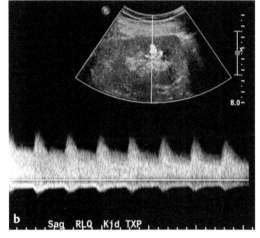

A.   Arteriovenous fistula.
B.   Pseudoaneurysm.
C.   Calculus.
D.   Renal vein thrombosis.

Answer:

A. Correct. The images demonstrate an area of color aliasing within the inferior pole of the transplanted kidney. Spectral Doppler demonstrates high-volume, low-resistance flow with arterial peaks. These findings are consistent with an arteriovenous fistula.

B. Incorrect. Pseudoaneurysms typically demonstrate a yin yang appearance on color Doppler images. On spectral Doppler, there is typically alternating flow above and below the baseline.

C. Incorrect. The "twinkle sign" may be observed with renal calculi and may demonstrate an appearance similar to the color Doppler picture. However, the flow pattern present on spectral Doppler in this patient confirms authentic flow as opposed to artifact.

D. Incorrect. Renal venous thrombosis typically results in reversal of arterial diastolic flow which is not present in this case.

Question 4.6: The images demonstrate an area of color aliasing within the inferior pole of the transplanted kidney. Spectral Doppler demonstrates high-volume, low-resistance flow with arterial peaks. Appropriate initial management of the finding would include?

A. Embolization.

B. Injection of sclerosant.

C. Expectant, as this is typically self-limiting.

D. Percutaneous nephrostomy.

Answer:

C. Correct. Iatrogenic arteriovenous fistulas are usually self-limiting.

A, B—Incorrect. The condition is self-limiting.

D. Incorrect. This would be inappropriate as there is no evidence of hydronephrosis.

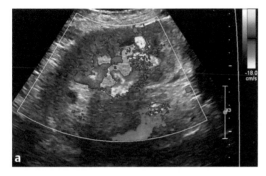

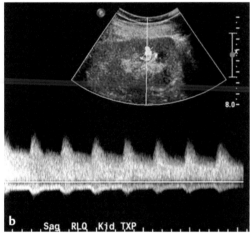

Question 4.7: What is the most likely diagnosis in this adult patient?

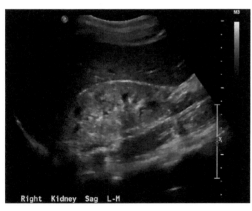

A. Autosomal recessive polycystic kidney disease.

B. Lupus nephritis.

C. Normal variant.

D. Acute pyelonephritis.

Answer:

B. Correct. The kidneys are usually affected in patient with systemic lupus erythematosus. The pathogenesis includes immune complex deposition within glomeruli. Typically, the kidneys demonstrate diffusely increased echogenicity.

A. Incorrect. Autosomal recessive polycystic kidney disease most commonly results in fetal demise. However, when presenting in childhood or adulthood, the kidneys are noted to be enlarged, containing innumerable tiny cysts.

C. Incorrect. This appearance is abnormal in an adult patient.

D. Incorrect. The renal sonogram is typically normal in cases of acute pyelonephritis.

Question 4.8: What is the most likely diagnosis in this adult patient?

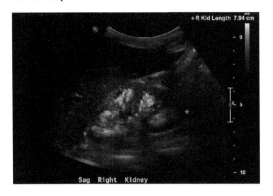

A. Autosomal recessive polycystic kidney disease.
B. Lupus nephritis.
C. Medullary sponge kidney.
D. Pyelonephritis.

Answer:

C. Correct. Medullary sponge kidney is the result of structural abnormality of the collecting tubules. The tubules become ectatic and serve as a point of calculus formation. This is a classic cause of medullary nephrocalcinosis and typically manifests as increased echogenicity of renal medulla.

A. Incorrect. Autosomal recessive polycystic kidney disease most commonly results in fetal demise. However, when presenting in childhood or adulthood, the kidneys are noted be enlarged containing innumerable tiny cysts.

B. Incorrect. The renal cortex is typically hyperechoic in lupus nephritis.

D. Incorrect. The renal sonogram is typically normal in cases of acute pyelonephritis.

Question 4.9: A transplanted kidney is demonstrated below. What is the diagnosis?

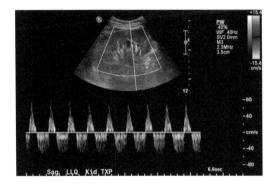

A. Arteriovenous fistula.
B. Pseudoaneurysm.
C. Calculus.
D. Renal vein thrombosis.

Answer:

D. Correct. The spectral waveform demonstrates reversal of arterial diastolic flow. In a transplanted kidney, this is the typical finding in renal vein thrombosis.

A. Incorrect. In the setting of an arteriovenous fistula, spectral Doppler demonstrates high-volume, low-resistance flow with arterial peaks.

B. Incorrect. While spectral Doppler may demonstrate alternating flow above and below the baseline within the neck of a pseudoaneurysm, the typical yin yang appearance of the actually pseudoaneurysm is not present on the color Doppler images.

C. Incorrect. A calculus is not imaged.

Question 4.10: The spectral waveform obtained in this transplanted kidney is presented below, demonstrating reversal of arterial diastolic flow. This finding is typical of renal vein thrombosis. When does this typically occur?

A. Within the first week post transplant.

B. Between 1 to 6 months post transplant.

C. Between 6 to 12 months post transplant.

D. After a year post transplant.

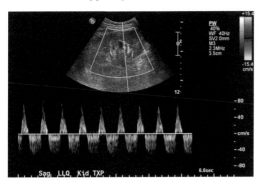

Answer:

A. Correct. Renal vein thrombosis typically occurs within the first week after transplantation and may be due to local compression from post op fluid collections, hypovolemia and surgical technique.

B, C, D–Incorrect. Renal vein thrombosis typically occurs within the first week after transplantation.

Question 4.11: The lower poles of this patient's kidneys have been repetitively difficult to demonstrate sonographically. What is the most likely cause?

Answer:

B. Correct. One of the most consistent sonographic findings in horseshoe kidney is the inability to adequately demonstrate the lower poles as they deviate medially.

A. Incorrect. Bowel gas would probably not be a repetitive problem in the same area. Also altering the patient's position and employing different degrees of inspiration would facilitate better viewing of the lower poles.

C. Incorrect. Shadowing calculi would be expected to produce echogenic foci with posterior shadowing, which is not present in this case.

D. Incorrect. Rib shadows originate from the body wall, closer to the near-field, which is not the case in this patient.

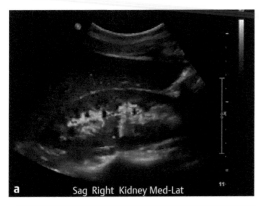

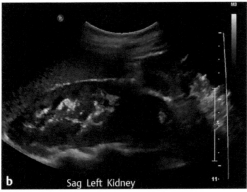

A. Too much overlying bowel gas.

B. Horseshoe kidney.

C. Multiple shadowing calculi.

D. Lumbar ribs.

Question 4.12: What anatomic structure is indicated by the *arrow*?

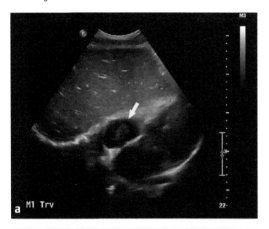

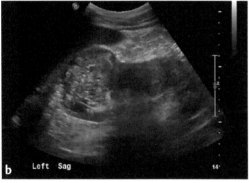

A. Gallbladder.

B. Pylorus.

C. Right atrium.

D. Esophagus.

Answer:

C. Correct. The *arrow* points to the right atrium.

A, B, D—Incorrect. These anatomic structures are not indicated by the *arrow*.

Question 4.13: At least what T stage of disease do the images in (Question 4.12) reveal, using the TNM classification?

A. T4.

B. T3C.

C. T3B.

D. T3A.

Answer:

B. Correct. The images demonstrate a rounded mass at the superior aspect of the left kidney with soft tissue material extending to involve the right atrium. These findings are typical of renal cell carcinoma with tumor thrombus extending to the right atrium, that is, above the diaphragm and hence the stage is T3C.

A. Incorrect. Stage T4 represents tumors that have spread beyond Gerota's fascia.

C. Incorrect. Stage T3B represents cases with tumor thrombus extending within the inferior vena cava but remaining below the diaphragm.

D. Incorrect. Stage T3A represents cases in which the tumor involves the adjacent perinephric fat or adrenal gland.

Question 4.14: This patient likely suffers from which of the following?

A. Essential hypertension.

B. Absence seizures.

C. Type 2 diabetes.

D. Bipolar disorder.

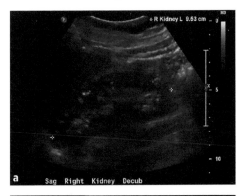

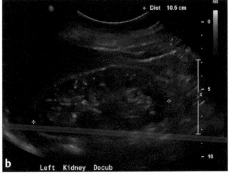

Answer:

D. Correct. The kidneys demonstrate multiple punctate echogenic foci throughout the parenchyma. These are typical findings of lithium nephropathy and thought to correspond to multiple microcysts throughout the kidney. Lithium is used in the treatment of bipolar disorder.

A, B, C—Incorrect. The findings are due to long-term lithium use.

Question 4.15: This adult patient presents with hematuria. Bilateral renal sonograms are obtained. Which statement is correct?

A. There is a contour deforming renal mass.

B. There is left upper pole caliectasis.

C. There is evidence of right renal artery stenosis.

D. There is no discernible cause for hematuria on the images provided.

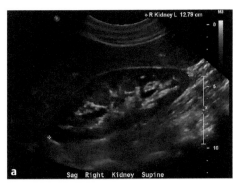

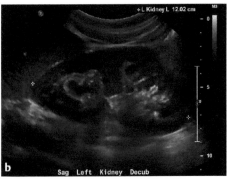

Answer:

B. Correct. Not only is there left upper pole caliectasis, there is also subtle soft tissue material within the calyx. This represents a urothelial neoplasm and the appearance is often termed an "oncocalyx."

A. Incorrect. No contour deforming mass is present.

C. Incorrect. Renal artery stenosis often presents morphologically as uniformly small kidney. Both kidneys are similar in size.

D. Incorrect. Left upper pole "oncocalyx" is present.

Question 4.16: What underlying condition should be excluded?

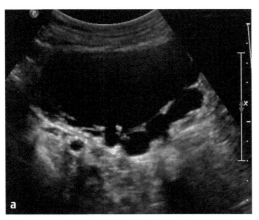

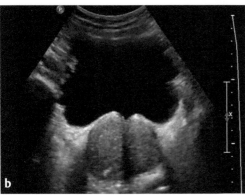

A. Prostate cancer.

B. Ectopic ureter.

C. Hydronephrosis.

D. Renal cell carcinoma.

Answer:

C. Correct. The images demonstrate bladder trabeculation and an enlarged prostate. The findings are consistent with chronic bladder outlet obstruction necessitating the exclusion of obstructive nephropathy.

A. Incorrect. There is no finding to suggest underlying prostate cancer.

B. Incorrect. There is no finding to suggest underlying ectopic ureter.

D. Incorrect. There is no finding to suggest underlying renal cell cancer.

Question 4.17: What is the cause of pain in this 35-year-old female?

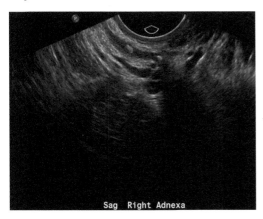

A. Acute appendicitis.

B. Distal ureteral calculi.

C. Ovarian vein thrombosis.

D. Endometriosis.

Answer:

B. Correct. The transvaginal sonogram demonstrates tiny echogenic calculi within the distal ureters (seen in the near-field), a useful albeit fortuitous finding in this patient.

A. Incorrect. The appendix is not imaged.

C. Incorrect. In this image ovarian vein thrombosis is not present.

D. Incorrect. Findings of endometriosis are not imaged.

Question 4.18: This new transplant requires which of the following options?

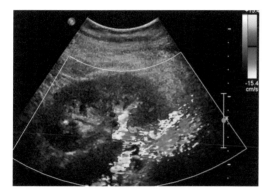

A.   Reexploration.
B.   Short interval repeat scanning.
C.   A nephrostomy tube.
D.   Urgent pelvic CT with intravenous contrast.

Answer:
A. **Correct**. The image demonstrates diminished perfusion in the upper pole of the transplanted kidney. This was due to acute occlusion of the upper pole branch of an early bifurcating transplant artery. This was successfully treated with open embolectomy.

B. Incorrect. This would not be helpful and the delay in definitive treatment would further compromise the graft.

C. Incorrect. There is no hydronephrosis.

D. Incorrect. The renal transplant vasculature is adequately evaluated with ultrasound.

Question 4.19: This diabetic patient presents with a history of abdominal pain and compromised renal function. What is the likely diagnosis?

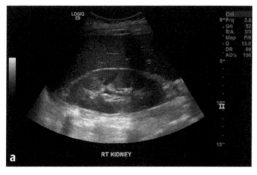

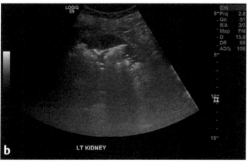

A.   Left nephrectomy.
B.   Medullary nephrocalcinosis.
C.   Xanthogranulomatous pyelonephritis.
D.   Emphysematous pyelonephritis.

Answer:
D. **Correct**. The left renal image demonstrates irregular echogenic areas within the renal bed with "dirty shadowing" consistent with renal parenchymal gas. In a diabetic patient, these findings are highly suggestive of emphysematous pyelonephritis.

A. Incorrect. There was no history of left nephrectomy.

B. Incorrect. This is not the appearance of medullary nephrocalcinosis which is characterized by increased echogenicity of the medullary pyramids.

C. Incorrect. This is not the sonographic appearance of xanthogranulomatous pyelonephritis which is characterized by an obstructing staghorn calculus within the pelvicalyceal system with hypoechoic, distended calyces.

Question 4.20: A 55-year-old male with a history of renal transplantation 6 years prior, presents with elevated creatinine. Sagittal views of the transplanted kidney are shown below, with color Doppler evaluation of a lesion. Which statement is correct?

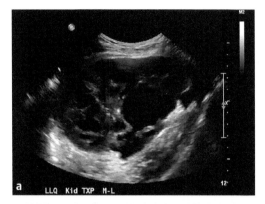

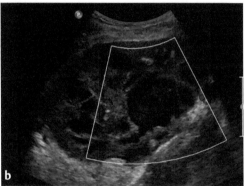

A. The images demonstrate multiple complex fluid collections likely representing abscesses.
B. The collections are likely to be sterile since renal transplants are not typically predisposed to parenchymal abscess formation due to the relatively short ureter.
C. The findings are consistent with lymphoceles.
D. The findings likely represent spontaneous intraparenchymal hemorrhage, a frequent complication of longstanding renal transplants.

Answer:

A. Correct. Recipients of renal transplantation typically experience frequent allograph infections due to immunosuppressive medications, frequent instrumentation, and indwelling catheters. Frequent glycosuria is also a risk factor. Prompt drainage and antibiotics administration is necessary to prevent loss of the transplant.

B. Incorrect. Transplanted kidneys are susceptible to infection.

C. Incorrect. Lymphoceles are typical anechoic and simple in appearance. Occasionally they may contain septations. Also, lymphoceles are usually external to the renal parenchyma.

D. Incorrect. Intraparenchymal hematomas usually result from interventions such as biopsies as opposed to being spontaneous.

Question 4.21: A 48-year-old patient presents for routine sonographic evaluation of her renal transplant. Transverse and sagittal images obtained during the evaluation are demonstrated below. What accounts for this appearance?

A. Mirror image artifact.

B. Transplantation of two kidneys.

C. Fluid collection.

D. Retained foreign body.

Answer:

B. Correct. The patient underwent en bloc transplantation of both kidneys from a pediatric donor. En bloc transplantation recipients show excellent long-term outcome, with 5-year graft survival similar to living-related donor kidneys.

A, C, D—Incorrect. The appearance is due to two separate kidneys.

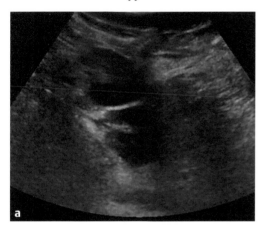

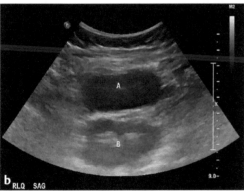

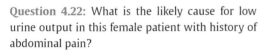

Question 4.22: What is the likely cause for low urine output in this female patient with history of abdominal pain?

A. Bladder leak.

B. Chronic renal failure.

C. Hypovolemia.

D. None of the above.

Answer:

D. Correct. The sonographic image demonstrates inadvertent malpositioning of the urethral catheter with the catheter balloon inflated within the vagina.

A. Incorrect. A bladder leak would manifest as pelvic free fluid.

B, C—Incorrect. The urethral catheter is malpositioned.

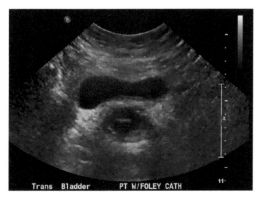

Question 4.23: What is the likely etiology of this fluid collection (*blue arrow*) in this diabetic male patient with a remote history of a renal transplant? The urinary bladder is indicated by the *yellow arrow*.

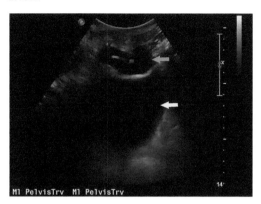

A. Urinoma.

B. Foreign body.

C. Abscess.

D. Artifact.

Answer:

B. Correct. This well-defined fluid-filled structure corresponds to the reservoir of a penile prosthesis device. Diabetic patients may suffer from erectile dysfunction as well as renal failure, thus this "fluid collection" should be entertained in men with renal transplantation.

A. Incorrect. Urinomas are uncommon and usually present early after transplantation.

C. Incorrect. An abscess typically presents as a complex fluid collection.

D. Incorrect. The well-defined fluid-filled structure corresponds to the reservoir of a penile prosthesis device.

Question 4.24: A left ureteral jet is observed. What accounts for this phenomenon?

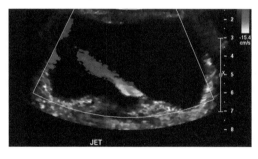

A. The Doppler shifts are mostly created by particulate debris within urine.

B. Differences in specific gravity between ureteral and bladder urine allow detection of the jet.

C. Changes in abdominal cavity pressure with respiration.

D. Changes in abdominal cavity pressure with Valsalva.

Answer:

B. Correct. Observed ureteral jets are at least partly due to the differences in specific gravity of "incoming" ureteral urine and long-standing urine within the bladder. Ureteral jets are less apparent if the bladder is quickly filled from empty, say by aggressive hydration, since the incoming ureteral urine and bladder urine would be in similar specific gravity.

A. Incorrect. Particulate debris may be seen in cases of urinary tract infections but does not account for ureteral jets.

C, D—Incorrect. These options does not account for ureteral jets.

Question 4.25: The right ureteral jet was not observed in this patient after 1 minute of continuous scanning. Which statement is correct?

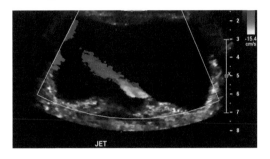

A. In the correct clinical context, an obstructing right ureteral calculus is likely present.

B. In the correct clinical context, a ureteral injury is likely present.

C. All of the above.

D. None of the above.

Answer:

D. Correct. None of the above. The rates at which ureteral jets are observed in normal volunteers vary greatly. One minute of observation is not sufficient to assume obstruction. Most protocols advocate for at least a 5-minute period of observation.

A, B, C—Incorrect. One minute of observation is not sufficient to assume ureteral obstruction. Most protocols advocate for at least a 5-minute period of observation.

Further Readings

Akbar SA, Jafri SZ, Amendola MA, Madrazo BL, Salem R, Bis KG. Complications of renal transplantation. Radiographics 2005;25(5):1335–1356

Baker SM, Middleton WD. Color Doppler sonography of ureteral jets in normal volunteers: importance of the relative specific gravity of urine in the ureter and bladder. AJR Am J Roentgenol 1992;159(4):773–775

Bent C, Fananapazir G, Tse G, et al. Graft arterial stenosis in kidney en bloc grafts from very small pediatric donors: incidence, timing, and role of ultrasound in screening. Am J Transplant 2015; 15(11):2940–2946

Cheng PM, Moin P, Dunn MD, Boswell WD, Duddalwar VA. What the radiologist needs to know about urolithiasis: part 1—pathogenesis, types, assessment, and variant anatomy. AJR Am J Roentgenol 2012;198(6):W540-7

Gosink BB, Leymaster CE. Ultrasonic determination of hepatomegaly. J Clin Ultrasound 1981;9(1):37–44

Coursey CA, Casalino DD, Remer EM, et al. ACR Appropriateness Criteria® acute onset flank pain—suspicion of stone disease. Ultrasound Q 2012; 28(3): 227–233

Cox IH, Erickson SJ, Foley WD, Dewire DM. Ureteric jets: evaluation of normal flow dynamics with color Doppler sonography. AJR Am J Roentgenol 1992;158(5):1051–1055

Dunmire B, Lee FC, Hsi RS, et al. Tools to improve the accuracy of kidney stone sizing with ultrasound. J Endourol 2015;29(2):147–152

Dunmire B, Harper JD, Cunitz BW, et al. Use of the acoustic shadow width to determine kidney stone size with ultrasound. J Urol 2016;195(1):171–177

Lalani TA, Kanne JP, Hatfield GA, Chen P. Imaging findings in systemic lupus erythematosus. Radiographics 2004; 24(4):1069–1086

Leder RA, Dunnick NR. Transitional cell carcinoma of the pelvicalices and ureter. AJR Am J Roentgenol 1990; 155(4):713–722

Ng CS, Wood CG, Silverman PM, Tannir NM, Tamboli P, Sandler CM. Renal cell carcinoma: diagnosis, staging, and surveillance. AJR Am J Roentgenol 2008;191(4):1220–1232

Ray AA, Ghiculete D, Pace KT, Honey RJ. Limitations to ultrasound in the detection and measurement of urinary tract calculi. Urology 2010;76(2):295–300

Strauss S, Dushnitsky T, Peer A, Manor H, Libson E, Lebensart PD. Sonographic features of horseshoe kidney: review of 34 patients. J Ultrasound Med 2000;19(1):27–31

Chapter 5

Hepatobiliary

Rashmi Nair and Adrian Dawkins

Questions and Answers

Question 5.1: What structure is indicated by the *arrow*?

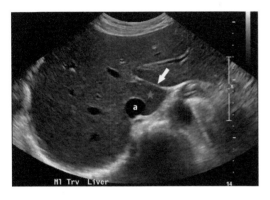

A. Falciform ligament.
B. Interlobar fissure.
C. Ligamentum venosum.
D. Gastrohepatic ligament.

Answer:

C. Correct. The *arrow* indicates the fissure for the ligamentum venosum. The caudate lobe is noted in close relation (*star*) abutting the inferior vena cava (IVC; a).

A. Incorrect. The falciform ligament runs in the plane between the medial and lateral segments of the left lobe of the liver. It is not imaged in this case.

B. Incorrect. The interlobar fissure runs in the plane between the right and left lobes of the liver. It is not imaged in this case.

D. Incorrect. The gastrohepatic ligament is not imaged. It forms part of the lesser omentum and connects the liver to the lesser curve of the stomach.

Question 5.2: What structure is indicated by the *arrow*?

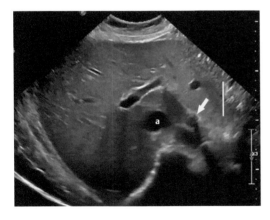

A. Gastroesophageal junction.
B. Cisterna chyli.
C. Aorta.
D. Lymph node.

Answer:

A. Correct. The gastroesophageal junction is often visualized on ultrasound imaging of the liver and is frequently confused with other structures. In the axial plane, it may be seen as a rounded structure to the left of the IVC (labeled *a*). If in doubt, the structure may be reviewed on a cine clip, allowing visualization of continuity above and below the diaphragm.

B. Incorrect. The cisterna chyli is a retrocrural structure related posteriorly and to the right of the aorta.

C. Incorrect. The aorta is not clearly imaged.

D. Incorrect. This does not have the typical reniform appearance of a lymph node.

Question 5.3: What structure is indicated by the *arrow*?

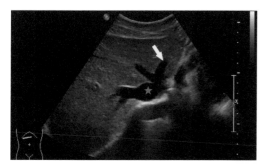

A.   Left hepatic vein.
B.   Recanalized paraumbilical vein.
C.   Left branch of the portal vein.
D.   Left gastric vein.

Answer:
A. Correct. The *arrow* indicates the left hepatic vein. The middle and right hepatic veins are also imaged, all three draining into the IVC (*star*). The classic appearance has been described as the "bunny sign."

B, C, D—Incorrect. These vessels are not imaged.

Question 5.4: What is the next appropriate step in imaging?

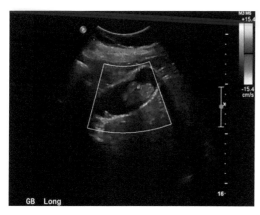

A.   Perform the Valsalva maneuver.
B.   Obtain spectral Doppler.
C.   Proceed to computed tomography (CT) with intravenous contrast.
D.   Proceed to magnetic resonance cholangiopancreatography with intravenous contrast.

Answer:
B. Correct. The image demonstrates a polypoid solid soft-tissue lesion arising within the gallbladder lumen. The color Doppler overlay demonstrates a tiny focus of color signal within the polyp. Because of the small size, this punctate focus should be reinterrogated with spectral Doppler to confirm authentic vascular flow as opposed to artifact.

A. Incorrect. The Valsalva maneuver would not be helpful.

C. Incorrect. While further cross-sectional imaging may provide useful information regarding local anatomy and distant disease, this is not the next appropriate step.

D. Incorrect. This option is not the next appropriate step due to the above mentioned reason.

Question 5.5: Polypoid gallbladder lesions greater than what dimension should be follow-up with repeat ultrasound?

A. 1 mm.

B. 4 mm.

C. 6 mm.

D. 10 mm.

Answer:

C. Correct. Gallbladder polyps are commonly encountered incidentally in daily practice. The vast majority of these polyps are benign and indeed nonneoplastic. At a size >6 mm, there is a slightly increased risk of an underlying adenoma which theoretically could progress to an adenocarcinoma. Consequently, polyps that are >6 mm in size warrant follow-up, where as those, ≤6 mm require no follow-up imaging.

A, B—Incorrect. Polyps >6 mm should be followed-up.

D. Incorrect. Some authors advocate for cholecystectomy for polyps exceeding 10 mm but this is debatable.

Question 5.6: The sonographic image below demonstrates a gallbladder mass in a patient with a known primary malignancy. What is the most common source of gallbladder metastases?

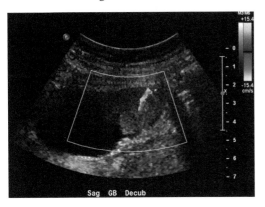

A. Gastric carcinoma.

B. Melanoma.

C. Renal cell carcinoma.

D. Hepatocellular carcinoma.

Answer:

B. Correct. Melanoma is reported to represent 60% of all gallbladder metastases in the western medical literature.

A. Incorrect. Although gastric carcinoma is a common source of gallbladder metastases in Asia, melanoma is a more common source in the west.

C. Incorrect. This is not the most common source of gallbladder metastases.

D. Incorrect. Hepatocellular carcinoma may directly invade the gallbladder, but is less likely to result in a true metastatic deposit.

Question 5.7: What is the likely diagnosis of the finding indicated by the *arrow*?

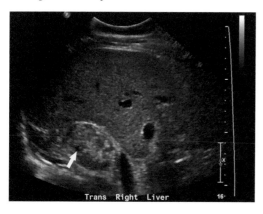

A. Hemangioma.
B. Hepatocellular carcinoma.
C. Focal nodular hyperplasia.
D. Myelolipoma.

Answer:

D. Correct. The image demonstrates a soft-tissue lesion in close relation to the right lobe of the liver. The lesion demonstrates echogenic (fatty) areas and is external to the liver parenchyma. The location and imaging features are consistent with an adrenal myelolipoma.

A, B, C—Incorrect. These options represents an intrahepatic lesion. The imaged lesion is extrahepatic.

Question 5.8: A 46-year-old male with a history of intravenous drug and alcohol abuse is admitted to the ICU with altered mental status. A sonographic image of his liver is presented below. Which of the following is the most helpful finding for the diagnosis of cirrhosis?

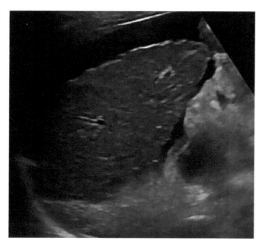

A. Diffusely increased liver echogenicity.
B. Heterogeneous liver parenchyma.
C. Liver surface nodularity.
D. Perihepatic fluid.

Answer:

C. Correct. Liver surface nodularity reflects the presence of regenerative nodules and fibrosis. This morphological feature is the most predictive indicator for the diagnosis of cirrhosis using conventional gray-scale ultrasound (US).

A. Incorrect. There are many pathologies that result in diffusely increased hepatic echogenicity and thus, this finding is not specific for cirrhosis. The common differential diagnoses include steatosis, cirrhosis, hepatitis, and chronic right heart failure. Diffusely increased liver echogenicity correlates more with hepatic fat content than fibrosis in cirrhosis.

B. Incorrect. There are several causes for liver parenchymal heterogeneity such as cirrhosis, infiltrating hepatocellular carcinoma (HCC), heterogeneous fatty deposition, and florid metastatic liver disease.

D. Incorrect. Perihepatic fluid is a nonspecific finding and may also be encountered in a variety of renal and cardiac diseases.

Question 5.9: The following US examination was performed on a 52-year-old male with chronic viral hepatitis. Which value should be reported?

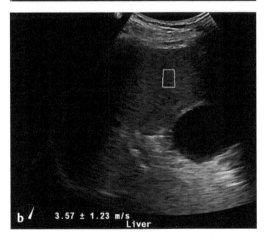

Abdominal	
— Abdomen stiffness —	
— Tissue stiffness —	
Stiffness Avg	[2.15] m/s
Stiffness Std	[0.46] m/s
Stiffness Med	[1.97] m/s
Sample 1	[3.00] m/s
2	[2.03] m/s
3	[2.30] m/s
4	[3.57] m/s
5	[1.19] m/s
6	[1.85] m/s
7	[2.04] m/s
8	[1.68] m/s
9	[1.90] m/s
10	[1.90] m/s

a

b   3.57 ± 1.23 m/s
Liver

A.   2.15 m/s.

B.   0.64 m/s.

C.   1.97 m/s.

D.   3.57 m/s.

Answer:

C. Correct. The patient is undergoing point shear wave elastography (pSWE). pSWE provides a measure of parenchymal elasticity which is used to predict the severity of hepatic fibrosis. Imaging is obtained via an intercostal approach, in a fasting patient lying supine or in the left lateral decubitus position. Ten acquisitions are obtained from the same general area avoiding large vessels and focal lesions. The median of these 10 measurements is to be reported. The obtained value correlates with the METAVIR liver biopsy score.

A. Incorrect. This value is the mean which is not the recommended value to be reported.

B. Incorrect. This is the standard deviation of the measurements and hence incorrect.

D. Incorrect. The highest obtained value is not the recommended value to be reported.

Question 5.10: What breathing instructions should patients be given during the acquisition of liver parenchymal elastography measurements?
A. Continue breathing gently during acquisition.
B. Take a deep breath and hold for acquisition.
C. Hold your breath for acquisition between episodes of quiet breathing.
D. Exhale forcefully, then hold for acquisition.

Answer:
C. Correct. A breath hold in between episodes of quiet breathing avoids wide fluctuations in hepatic venous pressure which may be encountered during deep inspiration or expiration. This in turn could influence the observed liver stiffness.

A, B, D—Incorrect. These choices could lead to erroneous measurements.

Question 5.11: All the following are indications for liver elastography except?
A. Chronic hepatitis C infection.
B. Nonalcoholic fatty liver disease (NAFLD).
C. Unexplained portal hypertension.
D. Acute hepatitis.

Answer:
D. Correct. Elastography plays no role in the work-up of acute hepatitis.

A. Incorrect. Chronic hepatitis C infection is an established indication for US elastography to assess the degree of fibrosis prior to the initiation of therapy and also for subsequent monitoring of the response to therapy.

B. Incorrect. Elastography is indicated for assessing the presence of fibrosis and assessing the risk of progression to cirrhosis in NAFLD.

C. Incorrect. Elastography is indicated in the work-up of unexplained portal hypertension to diagnose the presence of underlying cirrhosis.

Question 5.12: Two sonographic images are obtained in a patient with abdominal pain. What likely accounts for the echogenic lesion within the liver parenchyma?

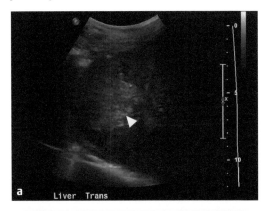

a Liver Trans

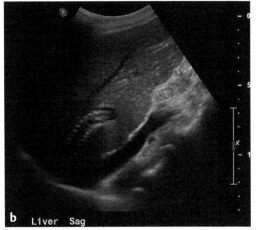

b Liver Sag

A. Hemangioma.
B. Hepatocellular carcinoma (HCC).
C. Focal nodular hyperplasia.
D. Hepatic adenoma with hemorrhage.

Answer:

B. Correct. The images demonstrate a somewhat ill-defined echogenic lesion (*arrowhead*) within a somewhat heterogenous liver. Also, the adjacent image demonstrates a transjugular intrahepatic portosystemic shunt (TIPSS). These findings indicate the underlying diagnosis of cirrhosis and an associated HCC. HCC can manifest in protean ways sonographically. Any large solid mass in a cirrhotic liver is HCC until proven otherwise.

A. Incorrect. While hemangiomas are typically echogenic, hemangiomas of this size are uncommon in the cirrhotic liver, presumably "consumed" by the cirrhotic process. The interpreting radiologist is duty bound to exclude HCC when these imaging appearances arise.

C. Incorrect. Focal nodular hyperplasia is a benign lesion of the liver, frequently possessing a central scar. It demonstrates a variable appearance on ultrasound and theoretically could account for the given appearance. However, an HCC is the much more likely choice.

D. Incorrect. Hepatic adenomas may be echogenic on ultrasound due to lipid content and associated hemorrhage. However, this is a much less likely choice, based on the given appearance.

Question 5.13: A 53-year-old male with hepatitis C, cirrhosis, and ascites presents for US. The following representative image was acquired. What is the diagnosis?

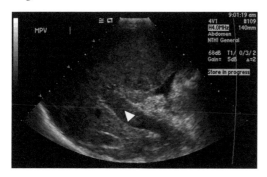

A. Cholangiocarcinoma.
B. Infiltrating HCC.
C. Metastases.
D. Regenerative nodule.

Answer:
B. Correct. The image demonstrates an expanded portal vein with isoechoic thrombus (*arrowhead*) contiguous with and similar in echotexture to the visualized abnormal liver. The findings are consistent with infiltrating HCC and associated "tumor thrombus." Doppler imaging may assist in demonstrating vascular flow within the thrombus, distinguishing it from bland thrombus which is commonly encountered in portal hypertension. Infiltrative HCCs account for 7 to 20% of HCCs and are seen almost exclusively in patients with established cirrhosis. This type of HCC can be very difficult to detect on imaging, especially with ultrasound. This pattern is important to recognize since ultrasound remains the primary modality for HCC surveillance.

A. Incorrect. Cholangiocarcinoma usually manifests sonographically as biliary dilation. A discrete mass is often difficult to detect.

C. Incorrect. Metastases typically tend to present as multiple lesions. It is uncommon for metastatic disease to present as an ill-defined mass with tumor thrombus.

D. Incorrect. Regenerative nodules are nonneoplastic and typically less than 2 cm.

Question 5.14: According to the American Association for Study of Liver Diseases (AASLD) guidelines, how often should patients at high risk for HCC be screened sonographically?
A. Every 3 months.
B. Every 6 months.
C. Annually.
D. Every 2 years.

Answer:
B. Correct. Patient at high risk for HCC should be screened every 6 months with US.

A, C, D—Incorrect. Screening should occur every 6 months.

Question 5.15: A 48-year-old female presents with pain and indigestion. She undergoes an US of her abdomen, representative images from which are demonstrated below. Of the options, which management strategy is most appropriate?

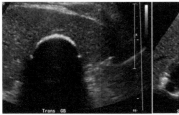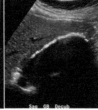

A. No follow-up required.
B. Follow-up with ultrasound in 6 months.
C. Cholecystectomy.
D. Hepatobiliary iminodiacetic acid (HIDA) scan.

Answer:

C. Correct. The images demonstrate a curvilinear echogenic focus arising from the wall of gallbladder with posterior acoustic shadowing. Indeed, a normal gallbladder wall is not perceived. These features are consistent with "porcelain gallbladder." While somewhat controversial, the 2 to 3% risk of gallbladder carcinoma in the setting of porcelain gallbladder usually prompts prophylactic cholecystectomy.

A, B—Incorrect. Prophylactic cholecystectomy is the most appropriate management strategy.

D. Incorrect. A HIDA scan would be inappropriate.

Question 5.16: The patient imaged below presents with abdominal pain. What is the likely underlying diagnosis?

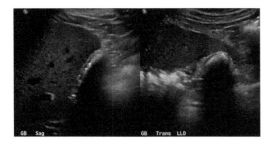

A. Porcelain gallbladder.
B. Emphysematous cholecystitis.
C. Cholelithiasis.
D. Pneumobilia and gallbladder luminal gas.

Answer:

C. Correct. The images demonstrate the classic wall–echo–shadow complex (WES sign). The sign is created by the gallbladder *wall* separated from the *echo* of calculi by intervening bile. The *shadow* is of course created by the calculi. Recognizing this sign is important as it may be mimicked by other entities such as loops of bowel or porcelain gallbladder.

A. Incorrect. Porcelain gallbladder represents calcification of the actual wall of the gallbladder.

B. Incorrect. Emphysematous cholecystitis is characterized by gas within the wall of the gallbladder.

D. Incorrect. Gas within the lumen of the gallbladder would result in the classic "dirty shadowing" appearance.

Question 5.17: A 62-year-old woman presents with right upper quadrant (RUQ) abdominal pain. A RUQ US is performed. What is the most likely diagnosis?

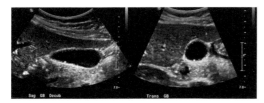

A. Inflammatory polyps.
B. Adenomyomatosis.
C. Cholesterol polyps.
D. Gallbladder carcinoma.

Answer:

C. Correct. A cholesterol polyp is the most common polypoid lesion encountered within the gallbladder accounting for 60 to 70% of lesions in some studies. As in this image, they appear as well-defined, round, echogenic intraluminal lesions attached to the gallbladder wall ("ball on a wall"). These lesions are situated within the wall of the gallbladder.

A. Incorrect. Inflammatory polyps typically occur in the setting of gallstones and chronic inflammation. They are typically multiple and <10 mm in size. Imaging features are nonspecific.

B. Incorrect. Adenomyomatosis typically presents as a focus of "comet tail" artifact arising from the gallbladder fundus. It represents cholesterol crystals with tiny intraluminal spaces (Rokitansky–Aschoff sinuses).

D. Incorrect. Gallbladder carcinoma is unlikely given the very small size and multitude of the lesions in this case.

Question 5.18: An ultrasound of the abdomen was performed in a 4-day-old neonate with vomiting and diarrhea. What is the most likely diagnosis in this child?

A. Necrotizing enterocolitis.
B. Portal vein thrombosis.
C. Budd–Chiari syndrome.
D. Acute hepatitis.

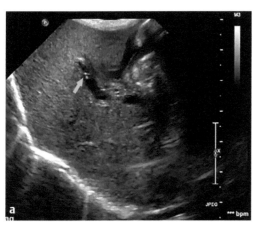

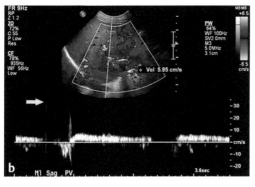

Answer:

A. Correct. The *green arrow* demonstrates echogenic foci with the portal vein, consistent with gas. This results in the bidirectional spikes seen on the Doppler spectral trace (*yellow arrow*). Portal venous gas is a key finding in necrotizing enterocolitis.

B. Incorrect. Flow is clearly demonstrated within the portal vein on color and spectral Doppler.

C. Incorrect. There are no presented findings in this case to support the diagnosis of Budd–Chiari syndrome, such as hypertrophy of the caudate lobe or occlusion of the hepatic veins.

D. Incorrect. There are no presented findings in this case to support the diagnosis of acute hepatitis, such as a swollen hypoechoic liver with echogenic portal triads (starry-sky pattern).

Question 5.19: A 54-year-old female with acute kidney injury undergoes a renal ultrasound. An incidental liver lesion is observed. What is the most likely diagnosis?

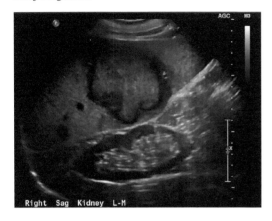

A. Abscess.
B. Focal nodular hyperplasia.
C. Hemangioma.
D. Metastasis.

Answer:
D. Correct. The sonographic image demonstrates a large isoechoic liver lesion with a surrounding hypoechoic rim. This represents the classic "halo sign" a frequently encountered feature of liver metastasis.

A. Incorrect. An abscess would present as a well-defined complex fluid collection possibly containing foci of gas and demonstrating peripheral hyperemia.

B. Incorrect. The halo sign is not typically associated with focal nodular hyperplasia.

C. Incorrect. Hemangiomas are typically hyperechoic with respect to normal liver parenchyma. Hemangiomas are not typically associated with the halo sign.

Question 5.20: The sonographic image below is obtained in a 64-year-old patient with abdominal pain. What other clinical sign or symptom is likely present?

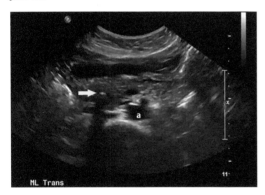

A. Absent or diminished bowel sound.
B. Jaundice.
C. Easy bruising.
D. Abdominal bruit on auscultation.

Answer:
B. Correct. This transverse view of the upper abdomen reveals a punctate echogenic finding with posterior shadowing within the vicinity of the pancreatic head (*arrow*). This represents a calculus within the distal common bile duct.

A, C—Incorrect. These symptoms are not typically related to the finding.

D. Incorrect. An abdominal bruit may be encountered in the setting of an abdominal aortic aneurysm, however the imaged aorta (*a*) is of normal caliber.

Question 5.21: A 44-year-old female with abnormal liver enzymes presents for routine RUQ ultrasound. A lesion is detected within the liver (*arrow*). Which statement is correct?

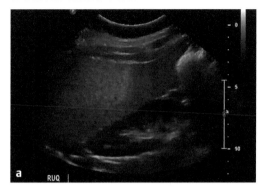

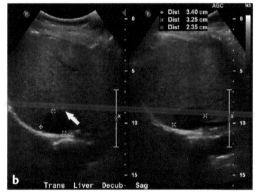

A. No further workup required as this finding likely represents fatty sparing in the setting of steatosis.

B. A targeted biopsy should be performed since malignancy is highly likely, given the appearances.

C. This lesion is unlikely to be a hemangioma given its hypoechoic appearance.

D. None of the above.

Answer:

D. Correct. Hemangiomas are typically well-defined and hyperechoic with respect to *normal* liver parenchyma on sonographic evaluation. However, in the setting of background hepatic steatosis, a hemangioma is frequently noted to be relatively hypoechoic.

A. Incorrect. Further imaging is required to help provide definitive characterization. Focal fatty sparing may present as hypoechoic areas within an otherwise echogenic liver, typically along the gallbladder fossa. However, the rounded appearance of this lesion as well as the location make focal fatty sparing less likely.

B. Incorrect. Definitive characterization should be attempted with magnetic resonance imaging (MRI) or CT with intravenous contrast prior to an invasive biopsy. This lesion was confirmed to be a hemangioma with MRI.

C. Incorrect. This option is not correct because of the reason mentioned above.

Further Readings

Barr RG, Ferraioli G, Palmeri ML, et al. Elastography assessment of liver fibrosis: Society of Radiologists in Ultrasound Consensus Conference Statement. Radiology 2015;276(3):845–861

Bloom CM, Langer B, Wilson SR. Role of US in the detection, characterization, and staging of cholangiocarcinoma. Radiographics 1999;19(5):1199–1218

Brancatelli G, Federle MP, Blachar A, Grazioli L. Hemangioma in the cirrhotic liver: diagnosis and natural history. Radiology 2001;219(1):69–74

Bruix J, Sherman M; American Association for the Study of Liver Diseases. Management of hepatocellular carcinoma: an update. Hepatology 2011;53(3):1020–1022

Colli A, Cocciolo M, Mumoli N, et al. Peripheral intrahepatic cholangiocarcinoma: ultrasound findings and differential diagnosis from hepatocellular carcinoma. Eur J Ultrasound 1998;7(2):93–99

Corwin MT, Siewert B, Sheiman RG, Kane RA. Incidentally detected gallbladder polyps: is follow-up necessary?—Long-term clinical and US analysis of 346 patients. Radiology 2011;258(1):277–282

Freeman MP, Vick CW, Taylor KJ, Carithers RL, Brewer WH. Regenerating nodules in cirrhosis: sonographic appearance with anatomic correlation. AJR Am J Roentgenol 1986;146(3):533–536

Gervaz P, Pak-art R, Nivatvongs S, Wolff BG, Larson D, Ringel S. Colorectal adenocarcinoma in cirrhotic patients. J Am Coll Surg 2003;196(6):874–879

Horowitz J, et al. ACR Appropriateness Criteria. Chronic Liver Disease—Diagnosing Liver Fibrosis. Available at: https://acsearch.acr.org/docs/3098416/Narrative

Jakate S, Yabes A, Giusto D, et al. Diffuse cirrhosis-like hepatocellular carcinoma: a clinically and radiographically undetected variant mimicking cirrhosis. Am J Surg Pathol 2010;34(7):935–941

Lafortune M, Trinh BC, Burns PN, et al. Air in the portal vein: sonographic and Doppler manifestations. Radiology 1991;180(3):667–670

Mathiesen UL, Franzén LE, Aselius H, et al. Increased liver echogenicity at ultrasound examination reflects degree of steatosis but not of fibrosis in asymptomatic patients with mild/moderate abnormalities of liver transaminases. Dig Liver Dis 2002;34(7):516–522

Mellnick VM, Menias CO, Sandrasegaran K, et al. Polypoid lesions of the gallbladder: disease spectrum with pathologic correlation. Radiographics 2015; 35(2): 387–399

Myung S-J, Yoon JH, Kim KM, et al. Diffuse infiltrative hepatocellular carcinomas in a hepatitis B-endemic area: diagnostic and therapeutic impediments. Hepatogastroenterology 2006;53(68):266–270

Reynolds AR, Furlan A, Fetzer DT, et al. Infiltrative hepatocellular carcinoma: what radiologists need to know. Radiographics 2015;35(2):371–386

Taylor KJ, Riely CA, Hammers L, et al. Quantitative US attenuation in normal liver and in patients with diffuse liver disease: importance of fat. Radiology 1986;160(1):65–71

Van Beers BE. Diagnosis of cholangiocarcinoma. HPB (Oxford) 2008;10(2):87–93

Wernecke K, Vassallo P, Bick U, Diederich S, Peters PE. The distinction between benign and malignant liver tumors on sonography: value of a hypoechoic halo. AJR Am J Roentgenol 1992;159(5):1005–1009

Yu NC, Chaudhari V, Raman SS, et al. CT and MRI improve detection of hepatocellular carcinoma, compared with ultrasound alone, in patients with cirrhosis. Clin Gastroenterol Hepatol 2011; 9(2):161–167

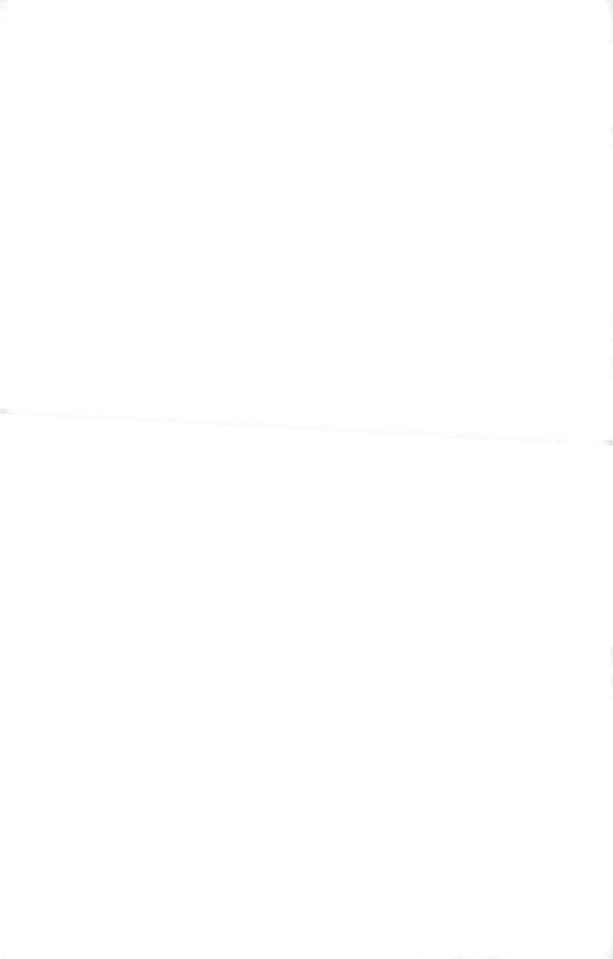

Chapter 6

Musculoskeletal

Paul J. Spicer

6 Questions and Answers

Refer to the following case for questions 6.1 to 6.3.

Case 1 A 48-year-old male has Achilles tendon pain. A single long axis (LAX) image of the Achilles tendon is provided. The tendon is noted by the *star* in the image.

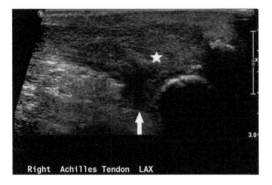

Right Achilles Tendon LAX

Question 6.1 What is the most appropriate diagnosis for the appearance of this tendon?
A. Normal tendon.
B. Tendinosis.
C. Partial-thickness tear.
D. Intrasubstance tear.
E. Full-thickness tear.

Question 6.2 What additional finding is noted on the image, annotated with a vertical *arrow*, which is often associated with pain?
A. Retrocalcaneal bursitis.
B. Subcutaneous calcaneal bursitis.
C. Calcium hydroxyapatite crystals.
D. Calcium pyrophosphate crystals.
E. Monosodium urate crystals.

Question 6.3: The patient requests an Achilles tendon injection for symptom relief and potential expedite healing. Options of corticosteroid injection and platelet-rich plasma (PRP) injection are discussed. Which of the following options best describes the appropriate site of injection?
A. Corticosteroid—peritendinous, PRP—intratendinous.
B. Corticosteroid—peritendinous, PRP—peritendinous.
C. Corticosteroid—intratendinous, PRP—intratendinous.
D. Corticosteroid—intratendinous, PRP—peritendinous.
E. Corticosteroid and PRP may be injected either intratendinous or peritendinous.

Answer 6.1:
B. Correct. The single long axis image depicts the Achilles tendon immediately deep to the skin surface, as annotated by the *star*. The echogenic shadowing structure along the right side of the image is the calcaneus at the tendon insertion. The image demonstrates thickening and hypoechogenicity of the tendon. This appearance is typical of tendinosis. Within the tendon are fibrils, which are the thin hyperechoic lines visualized in length on long axis images. The individual fibrils of the tendon remain intact, without fiber disruption. Therefore, a tear is not visualized.

A. Incorrect. A normal tendon is a thin structure which is hyperechoic. On long axis images, the Achilles tendon is immediately deep to the skin surface. The tendon in this case is much thicker and more hypoechoic than normal, therefore it is not a normal tendon.

C. Incorrect. The fibrils within the tendon remain intact, therefore no tear is present. A partial-thickness tear would result in disruption of a portion of the fibrils on either the skin surface or the pre-Achilles fat pad side of the tendon.

D. Incorrect. The fibrils within the tendon remain intact, therefore no tear is present. An intrasubstance tear would result in disruption of the fibrils within the tendon but without extension to the skin surface side or pre-Achilles fat pad side of the tendon.

E. Incorrect. The fibrils within the tendon remain intact, therefore no tear is present. A full-thickness tear of the Achilles tendon results in a complete tear through the tendon with or without retraction.

Answer 6.2:
A. Correct. There is distention of the retrocalcaneal bursa in the provided image, as annotated by

the vertical *arrow*. This is noted immediately deep to the tendon and along the superior surface of the calcaneus. It is visualized as a rounded anechoic to hypoechoic structure in the center of the image. This bursa normally resides between the Achilles tendon and the calcaneus; however, when it is distended the bursa extends superior to the calcaneus.

B. Incorrect. Subcutaneous calcaneal bursitis is distention of the bursa located between the skin surface and the Achilles tendon, which is not present in this case.

C, D, E—Incorrect. Crystals are echogenic structures which may be within or outside of a tendon. No crystals are noted in this case.

Answer 6.3:

A. Correct. Corticosteroid injections for tendons, including the Achilles tendon, should be injected peritendinous. An intratendinous injection of corti-costeroids weakens the tendon and increases the potential of tendon rupture. Plasma-rich protein (PRP) injections, however, should be performed intratendinous. This is typically performed in conjunction with tenotomy, both of which have a positive effect on tendon healing. The PRP material is able to aid in healing if it is injected within the tendon.

B. Incorrect. PRP should be injected intratendinous, not peritendinous.

C. Incorrect. Corticosteroids should be injected peritendinous, not intratendinous.

D. Incorrect. Corticosteroids should be injected peritendinous, not intratendinous. PRP should be injected intratendinous, not peritendinous.

E. Incorrect. Corticosteroids should be injected peritendinous and PRP should be injected intratendinous, not vice versa.

Refer to the following case for questions 6.4 to 6.6.

Case 2 A 65-year-old woman has medial epicondyle pain of the elbow. Two consecutive LAX images of the medial epicondyle and common flexor tendons are provided. The flexor tendon is annotated with the downward *arrow* in both images.

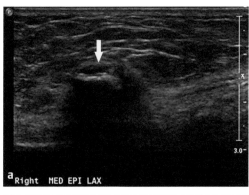

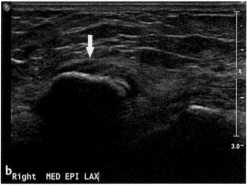

Question 6.4: What is the most appropriate diagnosis for the appearance of the tendon?
A. Normal tendon.
B. Tendinosis.
C. Tendinitis.
D. Intrasubstance tear.
E. Full-thickness tear.

Question 6.5: Which of the following changes at the tendon's cortical bone insertional site is associated with an abnormal tendon?
A. Increased concavity.
B. Volume loss.
C. Flattening.
D. Increased convexity.
E. Enthesophyte formation.

Question 6.6: The patient in this case requests percutaneous tenotomy for treatment. How does tenotomy help the healing process of a tendon?
A. Creates localized bleeding.
B. Creates neovascularity.
C. Creates enthesophyte formation.
D. Prevents fibroblast proliferation.
E. Prevents collagen formation.

Answer 6.4:

D. Correct. An intrasubstance tear is depicted in the ultrasound as anechoic or hypoechoic focal areas within the tendon. A tear leads to disruption of the echogenic fibrils within the tendon.

Intrasubstance tears remain localized within the substance of the tendon while the borders of the tendon on both the deep and superficial surface remain intact. In this case, the tendon which is immediately superficial to the shadowing cortex of the medial epicondyle and is annotated by the downward *arrow* has focal anechoic tears within the tendon. The deep and superficial surface of the tendon, however, are intact.

A. Incorrect. A normal tendon is hyperechoic with a fiber-like appearance or linear fibrillations within the tendon. This pattern is homogeneous throughout in a normal tendon. In this case, there are focal hypoechoic and anechoic areas within the tendon, suggesting the tendon is abnormal.

B. Incorrect. Tendinosis is depicted at ultrasound imaging as a thickened or swollen, and hypoechoic tendon. The echogenic fibrillations within the tendon remain intact and without a tear.

C. Incorrect. Tendinitis is not a term typically used to describe a tendon, because no acute inflammatory cells are noted within the tendon at biopsy. The term tendinosis is the preferred term.

E. Incorrect. Full-thickness tears are disruptions of the fibrils within the tendon along the superficial surface, the entire intrasubstance portion of the tendon, and the deep surface. The tendon may be retracted.

Answer 6.5:
E. Correct. Enthesophyte formation and irregularity of the cortex of the bone at the insertional site of the tendon often occurs in the setting of an abnormal tendon. This is best seen in image (**a**). The enthesophytes may intentionally be broken or scrapped during tenotomy to aid in the healing response.

A. Incorrect. Increased cortex concavity of the bone is not associated with tendon abnormalities. Focal

pitting or cystic change at the cortex is associated with tendon abnormalities, but the entire cortex does not undergo increased concavity in these cases.

B. Incorrect. Volume loss of the cortex is not associated with tendon abnormalities.

C. Incorrect. Flattening of the cortex of the bone insertional site does not occur, instead enthesophytes and irregularity of the cortex may occur in the setting of an abnormal tendon.

D. Incorrect. Increased cortex convexity of the bone is not associated with tendon abnormalities, instead enthesophytes and irregularity of the cortex may occur in the setting of an abnormal tendon.

Answer 6.6:
A. Correct. Percutaneous tenotomy is also referred to as fenestration or dry needling of a tendon. It helps elicit the healing response by encouraging localized bleeding that leads to fibroblast proliferation and ordered collagen formation. The hypoechoic portion of the tendon, as well as any anechoic cleft, is targeted. If neovascularity is present within the tendon it too is targeted. Tenotomy involves repeatedly passing the needle through the abnormal portions of the tendon to elicit localized bleeding within the tendon.

B. Incorrect. Tenotomy disrupts, not creates, neovascularity.

C. Incorrect. Enthesophytes may also be scrapped from the cortical surface of the bone during tenotomy. Tenotomy does not attempt to create enthesophyte formation.

D. Incorrect. Tenotomy encourages, does not prevents fibroblast proliferation.

E. Incorrect. Tenotomy encourages, does not prevents collagen formation.

Refer to the following case for questions 6.7 to 6.9.

Case 3 A 30-year-old male has the following images of his right supraspinatus tendon in the LAX (**a**) and short axis (SAX; **b**). The supraspinatus tendon is labeled by the *star* on the images.

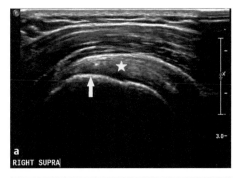

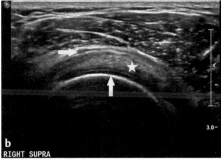

Question 6.7: What is noted by the vertical *arrow* on both the SAX and LAX images?
A. Greater tuberosity.
B. Lesser tuberosity.
C. Hyaline cartilage.
D. Fibrocartilage.
E. Subacromial-subdeltoid bursa.

Question 6.8: What is noted by the horizontal *arrow* on the SAX image?
A. Greater tuberosity.
B. Lesser tuberosity.
C. Hyaline cartilage.
D. Fibrocartilage.
E. Subacromial-subdeltoid bursa.

Question 6.9: These images were obtained using the modified Crass technique. The purpose of this technique is to bring the tendon out from underneath which structure?
A. Clavicle.
B. Coracoid.
C. Acromion.
D. Coracohumeral ligament.
E. Coracoacromial ligament.

Answer 6.7:
A. **Correct.** The greater tuberosity is the site of insertion of the supraspinatus, infraspinatus, and teres minor tendons. It is devoid of hyaline articular cartilage and the echogenic surface is the cortex of the greater tuberosity. It is labeled with the vertical *arrow* on both the LAX and SAX images.

B. Incorrect. The lesser tuberosity is the site of insertion of the subscapularis tendon. It is not included in the provided images.

C. Incorrect. The articular surface of the humerus and glenoid is lined by hyaline articular cartilage. The greater tuberosity, however, is not part of the articular surface of the humerus and is, therefore, devoid of hyaline articular cartilage.

D. Incorrect. The fibrocartilage structure within the shoulder joint is the glenoid labrum. It lines the glenoid and helps stabilize the glenohumeral joint. This is not associated with the greater tuberosity.

E. Incorrect. The subacromial-subdeltoid bursa is located on the image between the deltoid muscle and the supraspinatus tendon, labeled with a horizontal *arrow* on the SAX image. This is not associated with the greater tuberosity.

Answer 6.8:
E. **Correct.** The subacromial-subdeltoid bursa is located on the images between the deltoid muscle and the supraspinatus tendon, labeled with a horizontal *arrow* on the SAX image. It is not well visualized in normal individuals, seen as a thin anechoic structure between the deltoid and the tendon; however, in the case of bursitis it may become distended with fluid and is better appreciated. A distended bursa can also lead to subacromial impingement on dynamic maneuvers.

A. Incorrect. The greater tuberosity is the site of insertion of the supraspinatus, infraspinatus, and teres minor tendons. It is devoid of hyaline articular cartilage and the echogenic surface is the cortex of the greater tuberosity. It is labeled with the vertical *arrow* on both the LAX and SAX images. It is not associated with the subacromial-subdeltoid bursa.

B. Incorrect. The lesser tuberosity is the site of insertion of the subscapularis tendon. It is not included in the provided images.

C. Incorrect. The articular surface of the humerus and glenoid is lined by hyaline articular cartilage. This is not associated with the subacromial-subdeltoid bursa.

D. Incorrect. The fibrocartilage structure within the shoulder joint is the glenoid labrum. It lines the glenoid and helps stabilize the glenohumeral joint. This is not associated with the subacromial-subdeltoid bursa.

Answer 6.9:
C. Correct. The purpose of both the Crass and modified Crass techniques is to bring the supraspinatus and infraspinatus tendons out from under the acromion. The tendons normally reside beneath the acromion; however, the acromion obscures evaluation of the tendons in the resting position. By bringing the tendons out from under the acromion, the tendons can be visualized. This is done by either having the patient put their ipsilateral hand behind the back (Crass technique) or in their back pocket (modified Crass technique). These techniques are sometimes referred to as the Middleton technique.

A. Incorrect. The clavicle does not interfere with visualization of the rotator cuff tendons.

B. Incorrect. The coracoid may obscure a portion of the subscapularis tendon or muscle, but it does not obscure the supraspinatus or infraspinatus tendons.

D. Incorrect. The coracohumeral ligament does not obscure evaluation of the supraspinatus and infraspinatus tendons.

E. Incorrect. The coracoacromial ligament does not obscure evaluation of the supraspinatus and infraspinatus tendons. This ligament does reside superficial to the musculotendinous junction of the supraspinatus and infraspinatus tendons; however, the ultrasound beam is able to penetrate the ligament and therefore it does not obscure the underlying musculotendinous junctions.

Refer to the following case for questions 6.10 to 6.12.

Case 4 A 55-year-old male has shoulder pain. LAX and SAX images of the supraspinatus tendon are provided.

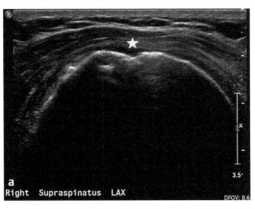

a
Right   Supraspinatus   LAX

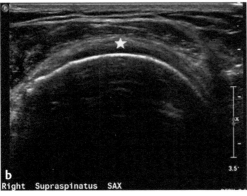

b
Right   Supraspinatus   SAX

Question 6.10: What is denoted by the structure labeled with the *star* on the above LAX and SAX images.
A.   Supraspinatus tendon.
B.   Infraspinatus tendon.
C.   Subscapularis tendon.
D.   Deltoid muscle.
E.   Biceps muscle.

Question 6.11: What is the most appropriate diagnosis for the appearance of the supraspinatus tendon?
A.   Normal tendon.
B.   Tendinosis.
C.   Partial-thickness articular-sided tear.
D.   Partial-thickness bursal-sided tear.
E.   Full-thickness tear.

Question 6.12: A 45-year-old patient presents with anterior shoulder pain. Which tendon is most likely affected?
A.   Supraspinatus.
B.   Infraspinatus.
C.   Teres minor.
D.   Short head of the biceps.
E.   Long head of the biceps.

Answer 6.10:
D. Correct. In the provided images, the supraspinatus and infraspinatus tendons are not visualized due to full-thickness, retracted tears. The *star* indicates the deltoid muscle which is occupying the space adjacent to the hyaline articular cartilage and the cortex of the humeral head

where the supraspinatus and infraspinatus tendons would normally reside if intact.

A. Incorrect. The supraspinatus tendon is torn and retracted. The stump of the tendon is not included in the provided images.

B. Incorrect. The infraspinatus tendon is torn and retracted. The stump of the tendon is not included in the provided images.

C. Incorrect. The subscapularis is not included in the provided images. The subscapularis tendon is best visualized with the lesser tuberosity externally rotated, however in this case, the greater tuberosity is shown on the provided images.

E. Incorrect. The biceps muscle is visualized overlying the humerus within the upper arm. The provided images are of the shoulder at the greater tuberosity.

Answer 6.11:

E. Correct. The supraspinatus tendon is not visualized on the provided images resulting from a full-thickness, retracted tendon tear. The stump of the tendon is not included on the images. Full-thickness tears result from a tear that extends from the bursal surface to the articular surface of the tendon. If the tear is also completely through the tendon from anterior to posterior, as noted on the SAX image, the stump may retract and therefore may not be visible on the images.

A. Incorrect. A normal tendon is hyperechoic. In the provided images, no supraspinatus tendon is visualized due to a full-thickness, retracted tear.

B. Incorrect. In tendinosis, the tendon swells or thickens, and becomes hypoechoic relative to a normal tendon. The tendon is intact. However, in the provided images, no supraspinatus tendon is visualized and therefore this is not compatible with tendinosis.

C, D—Incorrect. In partial-thickness tears, the tendon remains visible with a tear along the articular or bursal surface or within the substance of the tendon. No supraspinatus tendon is visualized in the provided images, therefore, this is not a partial-thickness tear.

Answer 6.12:

E. Correct. The long head of the biceps tendon is located in the anterior shoulder and is a common cause of pain leading to ultrasound examination of the shoulder. Pain may be the result of tendinosis, rupture, subluxation, or dislocation. The subscapularis tendon is the other anterior shoulder tendon and it too may be a source of pain.

A. Incorrect. The supraspinatus tendon and subacromial-subdeltoid bursa are part of the anterolateral shoulder ultrasound, and therefore are not associated with anterior shoulder pain.

B, C—Incorrect. The infraspinatus tendon and teres minor tendon are part of the posterior shoulder ultrasound examination, and therefore are not associated with anterior shoulder pain.

D. Incorrect. Examination of the short head of the biceps tendon is not part of the routine shoulder ultrasound. This tendon is also a less common cause of pain relative to the long head of the biceps tendon.

Refer to the following case for questions 6.13 to 6.15.

Case 5 A 45-year-old male has posterior elbow swelling and pain. Two images of the site of pain are provided.

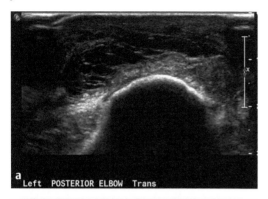

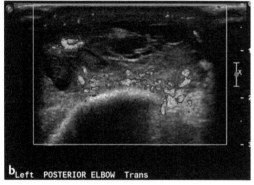

Question 6.13: Based on the provided images, what is the most likely diagnosis?
A. Cellulitis.
B. Myositis.
C. Bursitis.
D. Fasciitis.
E. Osteomyelitis.

Question 6.14: Which crystal disease would most likely be responsible for the imaging findings?
A. Calcium pyrophosphate.
B. Hydroxyapatite.
C. Amyloidosis.
D. Uric acid.
E. Oxalosis.

Question 6.15 Which elbow joint recess is the most sensitive location for identification of joint fluid?
A. Anterior coronoid fossa recess.
B. Anterior radial fossa recess.
C. Posterior olecranon fossa recess.
D. Annular joint recess.
E. Sacciform recess.

Answer 6.13:
C. Correct. The complex fluid-filled structure with surrounding hyperemia overlying the olecranon is the olecranon bursa. The olecranon is the shadowing structure within the middle of each image. Bursal distention of the olecranon bursa may be the result of trauma, infection, rheumatoid arthritis, or gout. In this example, the cause was infection of the bursa.

A. Incorrect. The skin and subcutaneous tissues overlying the olecranon bursae are not well-visualized due to the positioning of the focal zones. There is a subtle component of cellulitis, however this is not the predominant finding in this case.

B. Incorrect. Muscle is not clearly visible in this example. There is no evidence of myositis in this case.

D. Incorrect. Fascia is not clearly visible in this example. There is no evidence of fasciitis in this case.

E. Incorrect. The cortex of the olecranon is intact. There is no evidence of osteomyelitis in this example.

Answer 6.14:
D. Correct. Olecranon bursitis may occur as a result of uric acid deposition within the bursa in the setting of gout. The tophi within the bursa will be hyperechoic, which is not seen in this case since this example is the result of infection. Hyperemia and adjacent cortical erosions of the olecranon may additionally be noted.

A. Incorrect. Calcium pyrophosphate, also referred to as calcium pyrophosphate deposition disease (CPPD), does not typically involve the olecranon bursa. Instead, it typically involves the hyaline or fibrocartilage of joints such as the knee and wrist.

B. Incorrect. Hydroxyapatite, which often causes calcific tendinosis, does not typically involve the olecranon bursa.

C. Incorrect. Amyloidosis is not a crystal disease. Instead, it is deposition of a fibrous protein that can lead to amyloid arthropathy. It does not typically involve the olecranon bursa.

E. Incorrect. Oxalosis is the result of calcium oxalate supersaturation in the urine, which can in turn affect osseous structures. However, it does not typically involve the olecranon bursa.

Answer 6.15:
C. Correct. The most sensitive location to evaluate for joint fluid, or an effusion, is the posterior olecranon recess. When imaged in the sagittal plane,

superior and posterior displacement of the hyper-echoic fat pad will be noted.

A, B—Incorrect. The anterior recesses may distend with fluid in the setting of an effusion; however, these are not the most sensitive location.

D. Incorrect. The annular recess may distend with fluid in the setting of an effusion; however, this is not the most sensitive location.

E. Incorrect. The sacciform recess is an extension of the capsule of the elbow joint at the neck of the radius. This is not the most sensitive site for evaluation of joint fluid within the elbow.

Refer to the following case for questions 6.16 to 6.18.

Case 6 A 45-year-old female has a palpable finding on the palmar surface of her hand near the third digit metacarpophalangeal joint. SAX (**a**) and LAX images (**b**) are provided below.

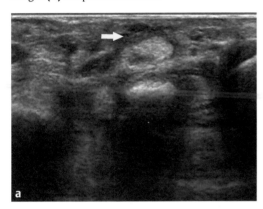

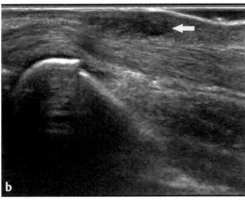

Question 6.16: Based on the provided images, what is the most likely diagnosis?
A.   Giant cell tumor of the tendon sheath.
B.   Dupuytren's contracture.
C.   Tenosynovitis.
D.   Ganglion.
E.   Foreign body granuloma.

Question 6.17: What does this diagnosis represent?
A.   It is thickening of the palmar aponeurosis.
B.   It is a soft-tissue reaction surrounding a foreign body.
C.   It is a localized form of pigmented villonodular tenosynovitis.
D.   It is synovial thickening within the tendon sheath.
E.   It is a cyst associated with trauma, degeneration, or idiopathic origin.

Question 6.18: Synovial hypertrophy and complex fluid within a joint may appear similar. Which of the following additional findings suggests a diagnosis of synovial hypertrophy instead of complex fluid within the joint?
A.   Joint recess compressibility.
B.   Increased blood flow on power Doppler.
C.   Redistribution of joint contents with transducer pressure.
D.   Hypoechoic appearance.
E.   Focally located within one joint recess.

Answer 6.16:

B. Correct. Dupuytren's contracture is the result of thickening of the palmar aponeurosis. The mass in the images, noted by the horizontal *arrows*, is in continuity with the palmar aponeurosis. This continuity is best seen on the SAX image as a thin, hypoechoic structure emanating from the mass. On ultrasound it will appear as an elongated, hypoechoic mass superficial to a flexor tendon sheath and without flow on color or power Doppler.

A. Incorrect. Giant cell tumor of the tendon sheath is a localized form of pigmented villonodular tenosynovitis. The mass is in contact with the tendon sheath, however the tendon is able to glide within the tendon sheath independent of the mass. This mass will have internal flow on color or power Doppler.

C. Incorrect. Tenosynovitis is abnormal fluid distention or synovial thickening within a tendon sheath. This may have increased vascularity on color or power Doppler.

D. Incorrect. A ganglion is a cystic structure. Ganglion are the most common masses of the hand and wrist and are benign. The most common location is along the dorsum of the wrist, adjacent to the scapholunate ligament.

E. Incorrect. A foreign body granuloma would have a foreign body within it, unless it has recently been removed. There is no echogenic foreign body within this mass. Also, foreign body granulomas will have increased vascularity on color or power Doppler.

Answer 6.17:
A. Correct. Thickening of the palmar aponeurosis is a description of Dupuytren's contracture.

B. Incorrect. Soft-tissue reaction surrounding a foreign body is the description of a foreign body granuloma.

C. Incorrect. A localized form of pigmented villonodular tenosynovitis is the description of a giant cell tumor of the tendon sheath.

D. Incorrect. Synovial thickening within the tendon sheath is the description of tenosynovitis.

E. Incorrect. A cyst associated with trauma, degeneration, or idiopathic origin is the description of a ganglion.

Answer 6.18:
B. Correct. Increased blood flow on power Doppler can be seen with synovial hypertrophy but is not usually seen within complex fluid.

A. Incorrect. Joint recess compressibility is typical of complex fluid. When compressed with the transducer, the fluid will compress away from the transducer, however synovial hypertrophy will not.

C. Incorrect. Redistribution of joint contents with transducer pressure is typical of complex fluid but is not seen in the setting of synovial hypertrophy. Similar to join recess compressibility, if pressure is applied with the transducer, the fluid can redistribute throughout the joint.

D. Incorrect. Both synovial hypertrophy and complex fluid may have a hypoechoic appearance.

E. Incorrect. Complex fluid may be focally located within one joint recess, however synovial hypertrophy is usually present throughout the joint.

Refer to the following case for questions 6.19 to 6.21.

Case 7 A 30-year-old female has ankle pain and a palpable mass. LAX (**a**) and SAX color Doppler images (**b**) are provided.

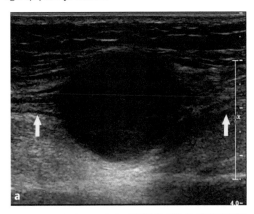

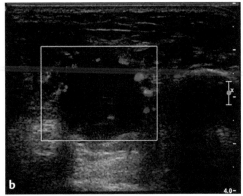

Question 6.19: Based on the images what is the most likely diagnosis?
A. Ganglion.
B. Lipoma.
C. Lymph node.
D. Soft-tissue sarcoma.
E. Nerve sheath tumor.

Question 6.20: What do the vertical *arrows* indicate?
A. Fat.
B. Muscle.
C. Vessel.
D. Nerve.
E. Fascia.

Question 6.21: What is the most common soft-tissue tumor?
A. Angiolipoma.
B. Lipoma.
C. Lipoblastoma.
D. Liposarcoma.
E. Hibernoma.

Answer 6.19:

E. Correct. A nerve sheath tumor is a solid soft-tissue mass that is in continuity with a peripheral nerve. These masses are typically hypoechoic and may have low-level internal echoes. They are round or oval and are well defined. The mass often will have increased through transmission, as this example does, which may cause it to be mistaken for a cyst. However, color or power Doppler imaging will demonstrate internal vascularity which will distinguish it from a cyst.

A. Incorrect. A ganglion is a cystic mass, however they will not have internal vascularity as the mass in this case does.

B. Incorrect. A lipoma may be present within the subcutaneous tissues or within a muscle. The echogenicity may vary depending on the location of the mass, either within the subcutaneous tissues or within a muscle, and the amount of fibrous tissue within the mass. Lipomas within a muscle or those which have more fibrous tissue will appear hyperechoic. The example in this case, however, is more hypoechoic and more round than is typical of a lipoma.

C. Incorrect. Lymph nodes are typically reniform in shape with a fatty echogenic hilum. Blood flow to the lymph node is usually through the hilum. The cortex is hypoechoic. The example in this case is not compatible with a normal lymph node.

D. Incorrect. Soft-tissue sarcomas are typically hypoechoic. They may have areas which are anechoic due to necrosis within the mass. They have increased vascularity on color or power Doppler imaging and have increased posterior through transmission. They, however, are not in continuity with a nerve.

Answer 6.20:

D. Correct. The vertical *arrows* point to the nerve as it enters and exits the mass. This is characteristic of a nerve sheath tumor.

A. Incorrect. The subcutaneous fat within the images is superficial to the mass.

B. Incorrect. No muscle is noted within the images.

C. Incorrect. Small vessels are noted within the color Doppler image; however, these are not depicted by the vertical *arrows*.

E. Incorrect. No fascia is noted within the images.

Answer 6.21:

B. Correct. Lipomas are the most common soft-tissue tumors, accounting for approximately 50% of all soft-tissue tumors. They occur most commonly in the fifth through seventh decades of life. They are composed of mature adipose tissue and they resemble subcutaneous fat. They may have a few thin septa, less than 2 mm in thickness.

A. Incorrect. Angiolipoma is a benign neoplasm which presents in the second or third decade of life as multiple, small, tender, subcutaneous nodules within the forearm, upper arm, or trunk.

C. Incorrect. Lipoblastoma is a rare neoplasm of childhood, typically occurring in children less than

3 years of age. They most commonly occur in the extremities as a painless, enlarging mass.

D. Incorrect. Liposarcomas account for approximately 17% of all soft-tissue sarcomas. They usually present in the sixth decade of life as a painless, enlarging mass.

E. Incorrect. Hibernoma is an uncommon benign tumor arising from brown fat. It presents as a painless, slow-growing mass in adults.

Refer to the following case for questions 6.22 to 6.24.

Case 8 A 55-year-old male undergoes an ultrasound-guided joint injection. A single image is provided.

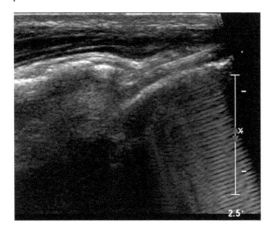

Question 6.22: What artifact is present in the image?
A. Beam width.
B. Reverberation.
C. Mirror image.
D. Refraction.
E. Increased through transmission.

Question 6.23: What would be the best way to improve this artifact?
A. Change the angle of insonation.
B. Adjust the focal zones.
C. Use color Doppler.
D. Increase the depth.
E. Increase the gain.

Question 6.24: What artifact is created when the ultrasound beam is angled as little as 5 degrees off perpendicular to the target?
A. Anisotropy.
B. Shadowing.
C. Ring-down.
D. Mirror image.
E. Beam width.

Answer 6.22:
B. Correct. Reverberation artifact occurs when two parallel highly reflective surfaces are present. The echoes may be reflected back and forth between the two surfaces before ultimately returning to the transducer. Since it takes longer for these echoes to return to the transducer, the ultrasound processor infers that they originated from a deeper location and places them accordingly deeper in the image. In this case, the two highly reflective parallel surfaces are the needle and the cortex of the bone.

A. Incorrect. The width of the ultrasound beam is initially the width of the transducer. However, as it nears the focal zones, the beam narrows and once it is distal to the focal zones it again widens, even wider than the width of the transducer itself. Beam width artifact occurs when the width of the beam is wider than the transducer. Echoes which originate from the portion of the beam that is beyond the width of the transducer are assumed to occur within the narrower transducer width of the beam and are placed within this portion of the image. This is why a large cyst may appear to have debris within the margins of the cyst if that portion of the cyst is outside the normal width of the beam.

C. Incorrect. In mirror image artifact, the primary beam encounters a highly reflective interface. The echo is reflected toward the transducer, however along its path it encounters the backside of a highly reflective surface causing the reflected echo to be reflected again toward the original highly reflected interface, away from the transducer. The original reflective interface again reflects the echo toward the transducer. This results in an image with a duplicated structure which is equidistant from and deep to the strongly reflective interface.

D. Incorrect. Refraction artifact occurs when the ultrasound beam travels through a medium other than human tissue, such as air or fluid. The speed of the ultrasound travels at a different rate in these other media, and therefore the echo is miscalculated and may be placed deeper in the image as a result.

E. Incorrect. Increased through transmission is the result of the ultrasound beam encountering a focal weak attenuating structure in the field. The amplitude of the beam that passed through this weak attenuating structure will be greater than the amplitude of the remainder of the beam in the image at the same depth. This increased amplitude is falsely recorded as increased echogenicity or increased through transmission.

Answer 6.23:

A. Correct. If the angle of insonation of the transducer is changed, or if the angle of the needle is changed, then the needle and cortex of the bone may no longer be parallel. Thus, the reverberation artifact would resolve.

B. Incorrect. Adjusting the focal zones would not resolve the reverberation artifact.

C. Incorrect. The use of color Doppler would not resolve the reverberation artifact.

D. Incorrect. Increasing the depth would not resolve the reverberation artifact.

E. Incorrect. Increasing the gain would not resolve the reverberation artifact.

Answer 6.24:

A. Correct. Anisotropy may occur when the ultrasound beam is angled relative to the target structure. This can occur when the beam is angled as little as 5 degrees. The result is normal tendons may appear hypoechoic due to the artifact, thus mimicking tendinosis. To determine if the hypoechoic appearance of a tendon is real or due to anisotropy artifact, the transducer angle can be altered by rocking the probe back and forth to see if the hypoechoic appearance of the tendon persists. If it does persist it is tendinosis, if not then it is the result of anisotropy artifact. A similar result of this artifact can occur with ligaments and muscle.

B. Incorrect. Shadowing occurs when the ultrasound beam is reflected. This results in an image with an anechoic region deep to the involved interface. This may also occur if the beam is absorbed or refracted. In musculoskeletal ultrasound, this may be encountered with bone, calcification, foreign bodies, or gas.

C. Incorrect. Ring-down artifact is a type of reverberation artifact in which the reflective echoes are more continuous deep to the source, usually the result of gas bubbles. The reflective echoes are tightly associated with each other and they produce an appearance of a continuous, echogenic stripe deep to the source.

D. Incorrect. In mirror image artifact, the primary beam encounters a highly reflective interface. The echo is reflected toward the transducer; however, along its path it encounters the backside of a highly reflective surface causing the reflected echo to be reflected again toward the original highly reflected interface, away from the transducer. The original reflective interface again reflects the echo toward the transducer. This results in an image with a duplicated structure which is equidistant from and deep to the strongly reflective interface.

E. Incorrect. Beam width artifact occurs when the width of the beam is wider than the target. Echoes originating from the portion of the beam that is beyond the width of the transducer are assumed to occur within the narrower transducer width of the beam and places them within this portion of the image. This is why a large cyst may appear to have debris within the margins of the cyst if that portion of the cyst is outside the normal width of the beam. Anisotropy artifact occurs when the ultrasound beam is angled as little as 5 degrees relative to the target structure. It may falsely make a normal tendon appear to have tendinosis. It may also make a normal ligament appear injured.

Further Readings

Burke CJ, Adler RS. Ultrasound-guided percutaneous tendon treatments. AJR Am J Roentgenol 2016; 207(3): 495–506

Feldman MK, Katyal S, Blackwood MSUS. US artifacts. Radiographics 2009;29(4):1179–1189

Gupta P, Potti TA, Wuertzer SD, Lenchik L, Pacholke DA. Spectrum of fat-containing soft-tissue masses at MR imaging: the common, the uncommon, the characteristic, and the sometimes confusing. Radiographics 2016;36(3):753–766

Jacobson JA. Fundamentals of Musculoskeletal Ultrasound. 2nd ed. Philadelphia, PA: Elsevier; 2013:2

Lee MH, Sheehan SE, Orwin JF, Lee KS. Comprehensive shoulder US examination: a standardized approach with multimodality correlation for common shoulder disease. Radiographics 2016;36(6):1606–1627

Chapter 7

Breast

Paul J. Spicer

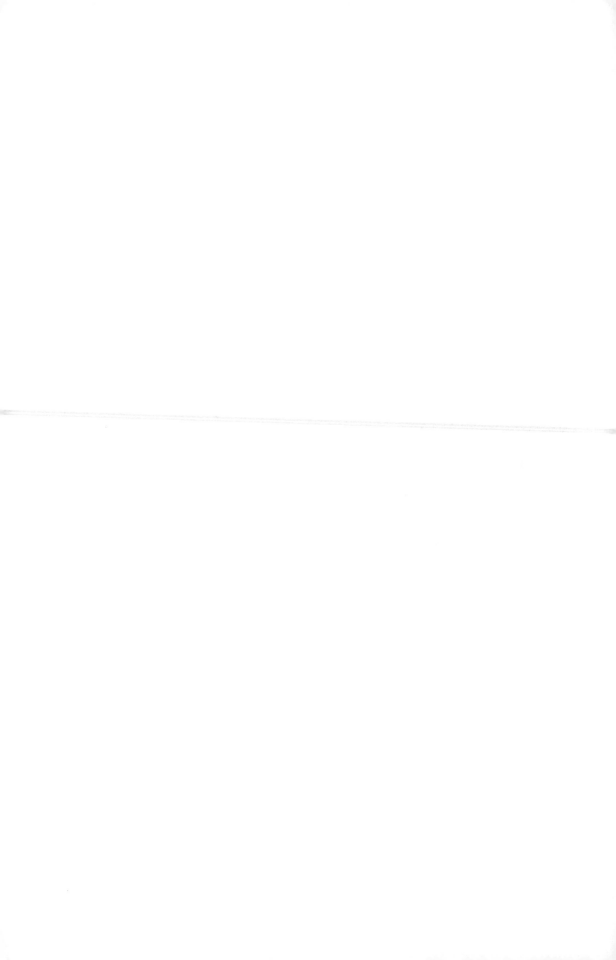

7 Questions and Answers

Refer to the following case for questions 7.1 to 7.3.

Case 1 A 45-year-old female has a palpable mass in her right breast. Radial and antiradial ultrasound images are provided.

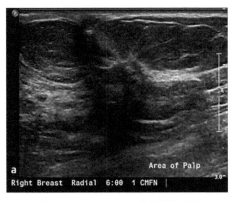

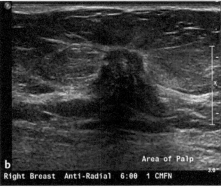

Question 7.1 Which of the following best describes the margin of the mass?
A. Irregular.
B. Indistinct.
C. Microlobulated.
D. Angular.
E. Spiculated.

Question 7.2: Which of the following best describes the shape of the mass?
A. Oval.
B. Round.
C. Irregular.
D. Microlobulated.
E. Angular.

Question 7.3: Which of the following features of a mass is most important for determining malignancy?
A. Shape.
B. Orientation.
C. Margin.
D. Echo pattern.
E. Posterior features.

Answer 7.1:
E. Correct. The margin of a mass is described as either circumscribed or not circumscribed. Circumscribed masses usually have an oval or round shape. Masses with margins which are not circumscribed have at least a portion of the margin which is not well-defined or sharply defined. These masses are further characterized as either indistinct, angular, microlobulated, or spiculated. The provided images depict a spiculated mass. Spiculated masses are those which have a margin with sharp lines radiating from the mass. This feature is often associated with malignancy. The spiculations are noted on both images as thin lines radiating from the mass.

A. Incorrect. Irregular is not an appropriate margin descriptor, instead it is a type of mass shape.

B. Incorrect. An indistinct margin is without a clear demarcation of at least a portion of the margin from the surrounding tissue. In the provided case, the margin is visible around the entirety of the mass.

C. Incorrect. An angular margin has sharp corners which often form acute angles. This is not present in the provided case.

D. Incorrect. A microlobulated margin has short cycle undulations, which is not present in the provided case.

Answer 7.2:
C. Correct. An irregular mass is a mass with a shape that cannot be described as either oval or round. This is typically a more worrisome finding for mass shape. The mass in the provided case is neither oval nor round.

A. Incorrect. Oval masses have a shape that is elliptical or egg-shaped. These masses may have two or three undulations. The mass in the provided case is not oval in shape.

B. Incorrect. Round masses have a spherical or circular shape where the anterior-posterior diameter equals the transverse diameter. This is an uncommon mass shape and does not reflect the mass in the provided case.

D. Incorrect. Microlobulated is a description of a mass margin, it is not a descriptor for a mass shape.

E. Incorrect. Angular is a description of a mass margin, it is not a descriptor for a mass shape.

Answer 7.3:

C. Correct. The margin of a mass is the most important feature for determining malignancy.

A. Incorrect. The shape of a mass is not the most important feature for determining malignancy.

B. Incorrect. Determining the benignity or malignancy of a mass based on orientation alone is discouraged.

D. Incorrect. The echo pattern of a mass alone has little predictive value for determining malignancy.

E. Incorrect. The posterior feature of a mass has more secondary value than primary predictive value for determining malignancy.

Refer to the following case for questions 7.4 to 7.6.

Case 2 A 50-year-old female has the following ultrasound images of a palpable mass in her left breast. She states the mass has not changed in size since she first noticed it several years prior.

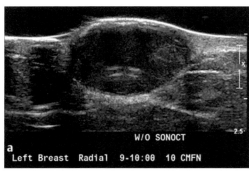

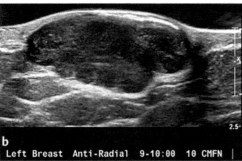

Question 7.4: What is the most likely diagnosis?
A. Complicated cyst.
B. Complex cystic and solid mass.
C. Skin mass.
D. Silicone granuloma.
E. Invasive ductal carcinoma.

Question 7.5: What is the most appropriate Breast Imaging Reporting and Database System (BI-RADS) assessment?
A. 2.
B. 3.
C. 4.
D. 5.
E. 6.

Question 7.6: What sonographic technique is applied in image (**b**) but not in (**a**)?
A. Spatial compounding.
B. Proper focal zone positioning.
C. Proper gray-scale gain.
D. Proper probe frequency.
E. Elastography.

Answer 7.4:

C. Correct. The mass is immediately below the skin surface and involves portions of the subcutaneous tissues, best noted by observing the edges of the mass. The mass is solid, without cystic components, and is oval in shape, parallel, with circumscribed margins. This is the appearance of a benign mass consistent with a large sebaceous cyst. A tract to the skin surface from the mass can be helpful for diagnosis as well, though not seen in this case.

A. Incorrect. The mass is solid, without any cystic components. A complicated cyst is a cyst that contains debris but does not have a solid component.

B. Incorrect. The mass is solid, without any cystic components. A complex cystic and solid mass has both cystic and solid components.

D. Incorrect. A silicone granuloma typically has the classic snowstorm shadowing created by the silicone. No shadowing is noted deep to this mass. Instead it has enhancement, meaning the area deep to the mass is more echogenic than the other tissue in the image at a comparable depth.

E. Incorrect. No suspicious features are noted with this mass to suggest malignancy.

Answer 7.5:
A. Correct. Skin masses are benign, therefore a BI-RADS 2 assessment is appropriate.

B. Incorrect. BI-RADS 3 assessments are for findings that have a less than or equal to 2% chance of malignancy. Since skin lesions are benign, this would be an inappropriate BI-RADS designation for this mass.

C. Incorrect. BI-RADS 4 assessments are for findings with a greater than 2% but less than 95% chance of malignancy. No suspicious features are noted and biopsy is not warranted. This is an inappropriate BI-RADS designation for this mass.

D. Incorrect. BI-RADS 5 assessments are for findings with a 95% or greater chance of malignancy. The mass in this case is benign, therefore this would be an incorrect designation.

E. Incorrect. BI-RADS 6 assessments are for biopsy-proven malignancies. This mass is benign in appearance and has not been biopsied, therefore this would be an incorrect designation.

Answer 7.6:
A. Correct. Spatial compounding is a technique used to improve resolution in the center of the image. This allows the margins of lesions to be visualized more clearly but the posterior features are less apparent. This is created by summing several overlapping ultrasound images obtained at different angles of insonation into a single image.

B. Incorrect. The focal zones are appropriately positioned in each image.

C. Incorrect. The gray-scale gain is appropriately set in both images. The gray-scale gain is set so that the normal breast parenchyma utilizes much of the gray-scale range.

D. Incorrect. The same probe frequency is utilized in both images.

E. Incorrect. Elastography was not utilized in either image. If strain elastography was utilized a color box would encompass the relevant finding, documenting the stiffness of the finding relative to normal tissue, and a corresponding scale would be noted in the upper-right-hand corner of the image.

Refer to the following case for questions 7.7 to 7.9.

Case 3 A 14-year-old female has a palpable abnormality in her right breast. Radial and antiradial ultrasound images are provided.

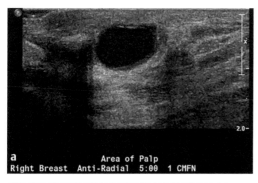

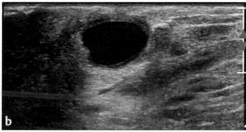

Question 7.7: What is the most likely diagnosis?
A. Simple cyst.
B. Clustered microcysts.
C. Complicated cyst.
D. Complex cystic and solid mass.
E. Lymph node.

Question 7.8: What is the posterior feature of this mass?
A. No posterior feature.
B. Twinkling.
C. Enhancement.
D. Shadowing.
E. Combined pattern.

Question 7.9: What type of probe does the American College of Radiology recommend for breast imaging?
A. Linear array, at least 10 MHz.
B. Curvilinear array, at least 10 MHz.
C. Linear array, at least 5 MHz.
D. Curvilinear array, at least 5 MHz.
E. Hockey stick probe.

Answer 7.7:
C. Correct. Complicated cysts are cysts which contain internal debris, as in this case. They do not have a solid component and have an imperceptible wall.

A. Incorrect. A simple cyst is a cyst that is circumscribed, round or oval, anechoic, and has posterior enhancement.

B. Incorrect. Clustered microcysts are a cluster of anechoic masses, each of which is less than 2 or 3 mm. They have intervening septations which are less than 0.5 mm in thickness. They do not have a solid component.

D. Incorrect. Complex cystic and solid masses have both anechoic cysts, or fluid, and echogenic solid components.

E. Incorrect. Lymph nodes typically have an echogenic fatty hilum and an outer cortex. They are reniform in shape.

Answer 7.8:
C. Correct. Enhancement occurs when the sound transmission is unimpeded as it passes through the mass, causing the area deep to the mass to be more echogenic than the adjacent tissue at the same depth. This is the posterior feature noted in this case. This is often seen with cysts, but some cancers also demonstrate this same pattern of posterior enhancement.

A. Incorrect. Masses with no posterior features are those in which the area deep to the mass is the same as the adjacent tissue at the same depth.

B. Incorrect. Twinkling is not a descriptive term used in breast imaging as defined by the BI-RADS atlas. This term is usually applied to renal calcifications.

D. Incorrect. Shadowing is noted when the area deep to the mass is attenuated relative to the adjacent tissue at the same depth. This can be seen in benign entities such as fibrosis, scar, fibrous mastopathy, and calcifications but it can also be seen in some cancers.

E. Incorrect. A combined pattern means the mass has more than one posterior feature.

Answer 7.9:
A. Correct. The American College of Radiology recommends the use of a broad bandwidth linear array transducer with a center frequency of at least 10 MHz.

B. Incorrect. Curvilinear probes are not typically used in breast imaging.

C. Incorrect. Frequencies of at least 10 MHz probes are preferred in breast imaging.

D. Incorrect. Curvilinear probes are not typically used in breast imaging.

E. Incorrect. Hockey stick probes are not typically used in breast imaging. These are more commonly used in areas where a smaller probe footprint is necessary such as in certain musculoskeletal situations.

Refer to the following case for questions 7.10 to 7.12.

Case 4 A 20-year-old female has a palpable mass in her right breast. Radial and antiradial ultrasound images are provided.

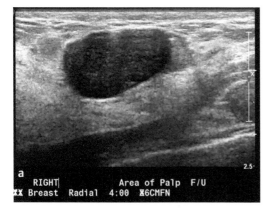

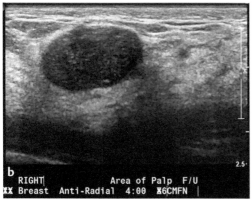

Question 7.10: What is the most likely diagnosis?
A. Simple cyst.
B. Complex cystic and solid mass.
C. Lymph node.
D. Fibroadenoma.
E. Epidermal inclusion cyst.

Question 7.11: What is the most appropriate BI-RADS assessment?
A. 2.
B. 3.
C. 4.
D. 5.
E. 6.

Question 7.12: How can it be determined if the depth of the provided image is appropriate?
A. The entirety of the target should be visualized.
B. The pectoralis muscle should be visualized.
C. The ribs should be visualized.
D. The pleura should be visualized.
E. The lung should be visualized.

Answer 7.10:
D. Correct. The images depict a solid mass with circumscribed margins, oval shape, hypoechoic to fat, minimal posterior enhancement, and parallel orientation. This is consistent with a fibroadenoma.

A. Incorrect. A simple cyst is a cyst that is circumscribed, round or oval, anechoic, and has posterior enhancement. The mass in this case is solid instead of cystic.

B. Incorrect. Complex cystic and solid masses have both anechoic cysts, or fluid, and echogenic solid components. No cystic components are noted in this case.

C. Incorrect. Lymph nodes typically have an echogenic fatty hilum and an outer cortex. They are reniform in shape. The mass in this case is not reniform in shape and an echogenic hilum is not visualized.

E. Incorrect. An epidermal inclusion cyst is a skin lesion. The mass in this case is within the breast parenchyma, not within the skin.

Answer 7.11:
B. Correct. In patients under 40 years of age, fibroadenomas with typical imaging features are given a BI-RADS 3 assessment.

A. Incorrect. A fibroadenoma can be given a BI-RADS 2 assessment if there are at least three total similar masses between both breasts, at least two in one breast, and at least one in the contralateral breast, or if the fibroadenoma has previously gone through a 2-year follow-up BI-RADS 3 cycle. Neither of these scenarios were noted in this case.

C, D—Incorrect. Masses in women under 40 years of age with typical imaging features of a fibroadenoma do not require biopsy.

E. Incorrect. This mass has not previously been biopsied, therefore it is not a biopsy-proven malignancy.

Answer 7.12:
B. Correct. The appropriate depth of an image is defined as including the breast tissue and the pectoralis muscle deep to it. By using this technique, it ensures that the entirety of the depth of the breast tissue is included in the image so that no breast lesions will be missed.

A. Incorrect. It is true that the entirety of the lesion should be visualized; however tissue deep to the lesion should also be visualized as well.

C. Incorrect. The ribs are deeper than what is required and therefore should not be included in the image.

D. Incorrect. The pleura is deeper than what is required and therefore should not be included in the image.

E. Incorrect. The lung is deeper than what is required and therefore should not be included in the image.

Refer to the following case for questions 7.13 to 7.15.

Case 5 A 54-year-old female has a palpable abnormality in her right breast. Radial and antiradial ultrasound images are provided.

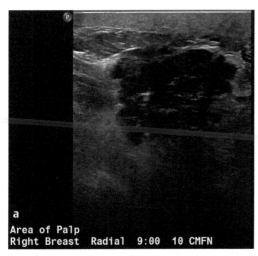

a
Area of Palp
Right Breast   Radial   9:00   10 CMFN

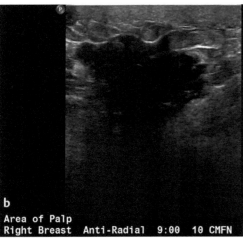

b
Area of Palp
Right Breast   Anti-Radial   9:00   10 CMFN

Question 7.13: What is the most likely diagnosis?
A. Complicated cyst.
B. Fibroadenoma.
C. Intramammary node.
D. Abscess.
E. Invasive ductal carcinoma.

Question 7.14: Which of the following additional findings is present in the ultrasound images?
A. Skin thickening.
B. Skin retraction.
C. Intraductal extension.
D. Ductal debris.
E. Vascularity.

Question 7.15: What skin thickness is characterized as skin thickening?
A. >1 mm.
B. >2 mm.
C. >3 mm.
D. >4 mm.
E. >5 mm.

Answer 7.13:
E. Correct. The mass is irregular in shape with microlobulated margins and adjacent architectural distortion of the Cooper ligaments. The features of the mass are worrisome for malignancy and biopsy is warranted. The biopsy results yielded an invasive ductal carcinoma.

A. Incorrect. The mass is solid, not cystic. Therefore, this is not a complicated cyst.

B. Incorrect. The mass has worrisome features and is inconsistent with a fibroadenoma.

C. Incorrect. The mass does not have the typical reniform shape as present in intramammary lymph nodes. Also, no fatty hilum is noted.

D. Incorrect. The mass is solid without cystic or fluid-filled areas, therefore this is not an abscess.

Answer 7.14:
A. Correct. Skin thickening is noted in the images. Skin thickening is defined as skin >2 mm in thickness. This is a case of inflammatory breast cancer resulting from an invasive ductal carcinoma with overlying skin thickening.

B. Incorrect. Skin retraction is noted when the surface of the skin is concave or ill-defined and is pulled in. Skin retraction is not present in this case.

C. Incorrect. Masses may have intraductal extension, where the mass extends into an adjacent duct. This often dilates the duct. Ductal extension is not present on the provided images.

D. Incorrect. Debris within a duct is typically a benign finding. Ducts are not visualized in the provided images, therefore ductal debris is not present in this case.

E. Incorrect. Vascularity is not detected in the provided images as color images were not included.

Answer 7.15

B. Correct. Skin thickening is defined as skin >2 mm in thickness. This may be diffuse or focal. The exception is in the inframammary fold or the periareolar region, where it may normally be up to 4 mm in thickness. Skin thickening may be seen in cellulitis, mastitis, or inflammatory breast cancer.

A. Incorrect. More than 1 mm is within the normal limits for skin thickness. Skin thickening is defined as skin >2 mm in thickness.

C, D, E—Incorrect. Skin thickening is defined as skin >2 mm in thickness.

Refer to the following case for questions 7.16 to 7.18.

Case 6 A patient with inflammatory breast cancer undergoes an ipsilateral axillary ultrasound. A single ultrasound image of one of the axillary lymph nodes is provided.

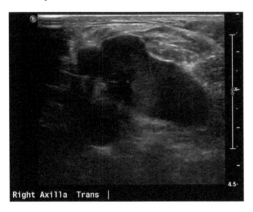

Question 7.16 Based on the ultrasound image, what is the next most appropriate step?
A. Nothing, the lymph node is normal.
B. Compare with the contralateral side with ultrasound to determine if the node is normal.
C. Compare with the mammogram to determine if the node is normal.
D. Recommend magnetic resonance imaging (MRI) to determine if the node is normal.
E. Recommend sampling of the node under ultrasound guidance.

Question 7.17 What cortical thickness is considered abnormal?
A. >1 mm.
B. >2 mm.
C. >3 mm.
D. >4 mm.
E. >5 mm.

Question 7.18: Which feature of an abnormal node has the highest positive predictive value for metastatic disease within an axillary lymph node?
A. Hilar blood flow.
B. Nonhilar blood flow.
C. Cortical thickening.
D. Calcifications in the node.
E. Loss of the fatty hilum.

Answer 7.16:

E. Correct. This lymph node is markedly abnormal. It has cortical thickening >3 mm with complete loss of the fatty hilum. This node should, therefore, be sampled under ultrasound guidance. This can be performed with fine needle aspiration (FNA) if cytopathology is available on site to analyze the specimen in real time to determine its adequacy. Otherwise, ultrasound-guided core biopsy could be performed.

A. Incorrect. The node is markedly abnormal in this case.

B. Incorrect. Comparing with the contralateral side is not necessary in this case as the node in question is markedly abnormal. Side-to-side comparison is sometimes helpful if there is suspicion of an inflammatory node resulting from a systemic disease.

C. Incorrect. Ultrasound is more sensitive and specific than mammography for evaluation of axillary lymph nodes.

D. Incorrect. Ultrasound is more sensitive and specific than MRI for evaluation of axillary lymph nodes. This node is obviously abnormal as per the ultrasound, therefore MRI would not add any value for evaluation of this node.

Answer 7.17:

C. Correct. A cortical thickness >3 mm is considered abnormal.

A, B, D, E—Incorrect. A cortical thickness >3 mm is considered abnormal.

Answer 7.18:

E. Correct. Loss of the fatty hilum has been reported to have a 100% positive predictive value for metastatic involvement of the lymph node.

A. Incorrect. Hilar blood flow describes the normal flow of blood to the lymph node through the hilum.

B. Incorrect. Nonhilar blood flow refers to flow of blood directly into the cortex of the node resulting from neovascularity, thus bypassing the normal flow through the hilum. This has a high positive predictive value for metastatic involvement, but it is less than 100%.

C. Incorrect. Cortical thickening is a suspicious finding, but it has a positive predictive value of less than 100%. It has a sensitivity of 88% and a specificity of 75%.

D. Incorrect. Calcifications in the lymph node may be a suspicious finding, particularly if the shape of the calcifications is suspicious. However, calcifications can also occur within lymph nodes from benign causes, such as the presence of tattoos in an area which drain to the axillary nodes.

Refer to the following case for 7.19 to 7.21.

Case 7 A 32-year-old female has spontaneous right bloody nipple discharge. Split screen image, including power Doppler, is provided.

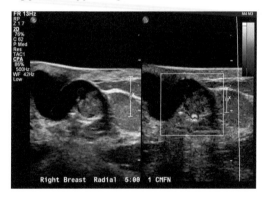

Question 7.19: The mass does not move with changing the positioning of the patient. What is the most likely diagnosis?
- **A.** Debris.
- **B.** Fibroadenoma.
- **C.** Papilloma.
- **D.** Invasive ductal carcinoma.
- **E.** Invasive lobular carcinoma.

Question 7.20: What BI-RADS assessment is appropriate based on the ultrasound image and history?
- **A.** 3.
- **B.** 4A.
- **C.** 4B.
- **D.** 4C.
- **E.** 5.

Question 7.21: Which feature of discharge is most worrisome?
- **A.** Bilateral, milky color.
- **B.** Unilateral, green color.
- **C.** Unilateral, milky color.
- **D.** Bilateral, green color.
- **E.** Unilateral, bloody color.

Answer 7.19:

C. Correct. The image depicts a solid mass with internal flow inside the duct. As per the history, this does not move with movement of the patient, therefore debris is unlikely. Debris also does not have an internal flow. The most common solid intraductal mass is a papilloma.

A. Incorrect. The finding is a solid mass with internal flow; therefore it is not likely to be debris. Debris does not have internal flow and it may move with changes in patient positioning, similar to sludge in the gallbladder. A technique called ballottement can also be used to differentiate debris from a solid mass. When pressure from the probe is applied to the area of concern, debris will disperse away from the pressure with ballottement while a solid mass will not.

B. Incorrect. The image does not have the typical features of a fibroadenoma.

D. Incorrect. The most common solid intraductal mass is a papilloma, not invasive ductal carcinoma.

E. Incorrect. The most common solid intraductal mass is a papilloma, not invasive lobular carcinoma.

Answer 7.20:

B. Correct. The correct BI-RADS assessment for the history and ultrasound image is 4A. Spontaneous bloody nipple discharge with an intraductal mass noted by ultrasound has a positive predictive value of malignancy of 8%. 4A findings have >2% but <10% chance of malignancy.

A. Incorrect. BI-RADS 3 findings have a less than 2% chance of malignancy. This finding, however, has an 8% chance of malignancy and is, therefore, a 4A finding.

C. Incorrect. BI-RADS 4B findings have a ≥10% but <50% chance of malignancy. This finding, however, only has an 8% chance of malignancy and is, therefore, a 4A finding.

D. Incorrect. BI-RADS 4C findings have a ≥50% but <95% chance of malignancy. This finding, however, only has an 8% chance of malignancy and is, therefore, a 4A finding.

E. Incorrect. BI-RADS 5 findings have a ≥95% chance of malignancy. This finding, however, only has an 8% chance of malignancy and is, therefore, a 4A finding.

Answer 7.21:

E. Correct. Worrisome features of malignancy include a discharge that is clear or bloody in color, unilateral, spontaneous, and via a single duct. Features that are less concerning include a discharge that is milky or yellow in color, bilateral, nonspontaneous, and via multiple ducts. The worrisome features collectively point to concern for a mass within a single ductal system within a breast which may be bleeding or generating clear fluid.

A. Incorrect. Both bilaterality and milky color are not typically worrisome findings.

B. Incorrect. Green color is not typically a worrisome finding.

C. Incorrect. Milky color is not typically a worrisome finding.

D. Incorrect. Both bilaterality and green color are not typically worrisome findings.

Refer to the following case for 7.22 to 7.24.

Case 8 A 55-year-old male has left breast tenderness and a palpable abnormality. Transverse and long axis ultrasound images are provided.

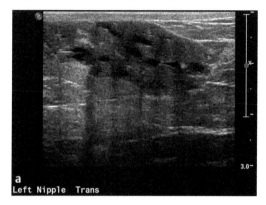

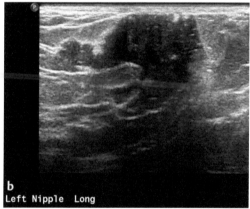

Question 7.22: What is the most likely diagnosis?
A. Gynecomastia.
B. Papilloma.
C. Fibroadenoma.
D. Ductal carcinoma in situ.
E. Invasive lobular carcinoma.

Question 7.23: What is the most appropriate BI-RADS assessment?
A. 2.
B. 3.
C. 4.
D. 5.
E. 6.

Question 7.24: A 40-year-old female has a mammogram and ultrasound depicting an abnormal axillary node which has previously been proven to represent lymphoma by biopsy. No other suspicious findings are noted. With this information, what is the appropriate BI-RADS assessment for the imaging findings in this case?
A. 2.
B. 3.
C. 4.
D. 5.
E. 6.

Answer 7.22:
A. Correct. The images depict gynecomastia in a male patient. No focal mass or suspicious abnormality is noted. Gynecomastia has the typical appearance of female breast tissue with ducts and stroma; however, no lobules are typically present. The ultrasound in this case has the usual depiction of stroma and ducts in the subareolar region of the breast.

B. Incorrect. No intraductal mass is noted.

C. Incorrect. No solid mass is noted. Males do not typically have lobules therefore they do not have masses that start in the lobule, such as a fibroadenoma.

D. Incorrect. No solid mass or intraductal mass is noted.

E. Incorrect. No solid mass is noted. Males do not typically have lobules therefore they do not have masses that start in the lobule, such as invasive lobular carcinoma.

Answer 7.23:
A. Correct. Gynecomastia is benign, therefore a BI-RADS 2 assessment is appropriate.

B. Incorrect. Gynecomastia is benign, therefore a BI-RADS 2 assessment is appropriate. BI-RADS 3 is for a finding which is probably benign but still has <2% chance of malignancy.

C. Incorrect. Gynecomastia is benign, therefore a BI-RADS 2 assessment is appropriate. BI-RADS 4 is for a finding which is suspicious.

D. Incorrect. Gynecomastia is benign, therefore a BI-RADS 2 assessment is appropriate. BI-RADS 5 is for a finding which is highly suggestive of malignancy.

E. Incorrect. Gynecomastia is benign, therefore a BI-RADS 2 assessment is appropriate. BI-RADS 6 is for a biopsy-proven malignancy.

Answer 7.24:

A. Correct. Though the patient has a malignancy, the malignancy is not breast related. The BI-RADS assessment only applies to breast cancer, therefore the patient in this case is given a BI-RADS 2 assessment for the breast findings instead of a BI-RADS 6 for biopsy-proven lymphoma.

B. Incorrect. The findings are benign, therefore follow-up as a BI-RADS 3 assessment if inappropriate.

C. Incorrect. The findings are benign, no breast finding is noted which requires biopsy under a BI-RADS 4 assessment.

D. Incorrect. The findings are benign, no breast findings are noted which requires a biopsy under a BI-RADS 5 assessment.

E. Incorrect. The patient does have lymphoma; however, it is not breast related therefore it is not considered in the BI-RADS assessment. The breast findings are benign, therefore a BI-RADS 2 assessment is given. It would be appropriate to add a sentence in the recommendations noting the presence of the abnormal node and that it is consistent with the known history of lymphoma.

Further Readings

Mainiero MB, Cinelli CM, Koelliker SL, Graves TA, Chung MA. Axillary ultrasound and fine-needle aspiration in the preoperative evaluation of the breast cancer patient: an algorithm based on tumor size and lymph node appearance. AJR Am J Roentgenol 2010;195(5):1261–1267

Mendelson EB, Böhm-Vélez M, Berg WA, et al. ACR BI-RADS® Ultrasound. In: ACR BI-RADS® Atlas, Breast Imaging Reporting and Data System. Reston, VA, American College of Radiology; 2013

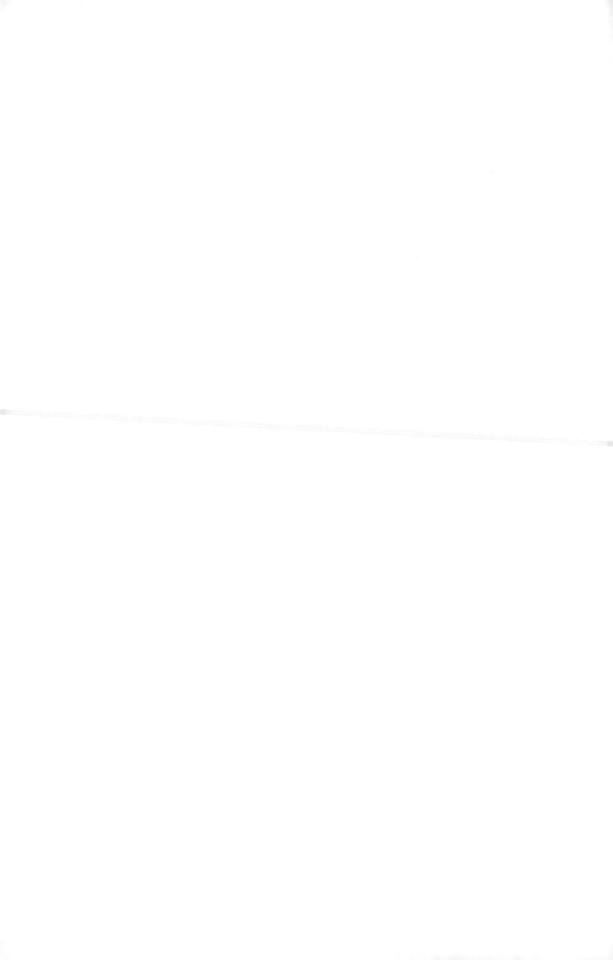

Chapter 8

Neck

Adrian Dawkins

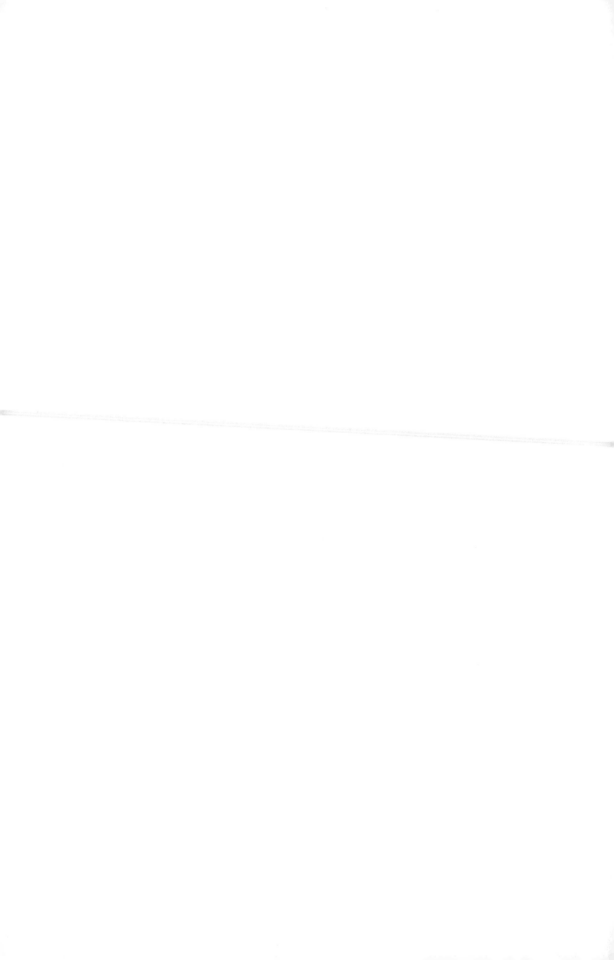

8 Questions and Answers

Refer to the following figure for questions 8.1 and 8.2.

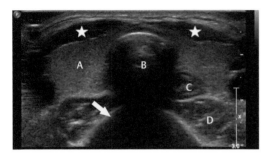

Question 8.1 This 35-year-old patient is scheduled for a barium swallow within the radiology department. During the study, the patient aspirates barium. Which structures will be opacified by barium?
A. A and B.
B. A and C.
C. B and C.
D. B and D.

Question 8.2: What frequency is typically employed in the sonographic evaluation of neck structures?
A. 2 to 3 MHz.
B. 3 to 5 MHz.
C. 5 to 12 MHz.
D. 30 to 35 MHz.

Answer 8.1:
C. Correct. This high-resolution sonographic image depicts a transverse view of the neck at the level of the thyroid gland. The butterfly-shaped thyroid gland is seen as a smooth fairly echogenic structure with right (A) and left lobes connected by the midline isthmus which is positioned anterior to the trachea (B). In the supine position, the esophagus (C) is frequently identified as a circular structure with several layers just the left and posterior to the trachea. The layered appearance of the esophagus is due to the differing echogenicities of wall components. The curved reflective surface of a cervical vertebral body (*yellow arrow*) is noted posterior to the trachea. Paired strap (*star*) and longus colli muscles (D) are also noted.

A. Incorrect. This represents the right lobe of the thyroid and trachea respectively.

B. Incorrect. This represents the right lobe of the thyroid and the esophagus respectively.

D. Incorrect. This represents the trachea and the longus colli muscle respectively.

Answer 8.2:
C. Correct. The superficial location of neck structures as well as large surface area of overlying skin, allow sonographic evaluation at high frequencies using a linear transducer. The resulting image is typically of high resolution, optimal for discerning anatomy and pathology, as well as guiding interventions.

A. Incorrect. This frequency range is typically employed for abdominopelvic scanning, particularly in obese patients, due to better penetration of the low frequency sound beam.

B. Incorrect. This frequency range is typically employed for abdominopelvic scanning.

D. Incorrect. This frequency range is not typically used in medical imaging.

Question 8.3: This image is obtained from a submental view of the neck. What structures are labeled A, B, and C?

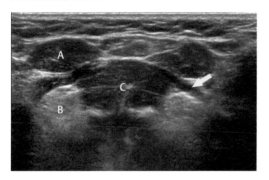

A. Mylohoid muscle, submandibular gland, and anterior belly of the diagastric muscle respectively.
B. Mylohoid muscle, submandibular gland, and the tongue respectively.
C. Anterior belly of the digastric muscle, sublingual gland, and the tongue respectively.
D. Anterior belly of the digastric muscle, submandibular gland, and the tongue respectively.

Answer:
C. Correct. The submental view is easily acquired by positioning the transducer in such a way that the footprint of the probe contacts the skin beneath the chin. The resulting image, when the probe is held transverse, is an "upside down coronal view" of the face. The anterior bellies of the digastric muscles (A) are seen as paired superficial structures. The mylohyoid muscle (*yellow arrow*) is seen as a superficial diaphragm-like muscle forming the floor of the mouth. Deep to this, the tongue is seen as a midline collection of several muscle bellies (C) with the echogenic sublingual glands (B) on either side. The image is classic and typically symmetric.

A. Incorrect. The mylohyoid muscle is indicated by the *yellow arrow*. The submandibular glands are not imaged. The anterior belly of the digastric muscle is indicated by (A).

B. Incorrect. The mylohyoid muscle is indicated by the *yellow arrow*. The submandibular glands are not imaged. The tongue is indicated by (C).

D. Incorrect. The anterior belly of the digastric muscle is indicated by (A). The submandibular glands are not imaged. The tongue is indicated by (C).

Question 8.4: The sonographic image below represents a longitudinal midline view of the neck. What structure is labeled A and B?

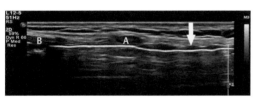

A. Thyroid cartilage and the thyroid isthmus.
B. Thyroid isthmus and the cricoid cartilage.
C. Thyroid cartilage and the cricoid cartilage.
D. Cricoid cartilage and a tracheal ring.

Answer:
C. Correct. This sonographic image is readily obtained by placing the transducer within the midline of the neck in the longitudinal plane. Ample ultrasound gel is required to maintain skin contact. The repetitive tracheal cartilaginous rings (*yellow arrow*) are noted as hypoechoic structures along the length of the trachea. The long slender echogenic line running along the trachea represents the highly reflective air that occupies the tracheal lumen. The cricoid cartilage is a larger, circumferentially complete cartilaginous ring at the cranial aspect of the trachea. The thyroid cartilage is seen as a larger hypoechoic structure at the cranial aspect of the image. The cricothyroid membrane occupies the space between the thyroid and cricoid cartilages and serves as the site for a cricothyroidotomy, an airway rescuing procedure.

A, B—Incorrect. The thyroid isthmus is not well-depicted but would be expected to be hyperechoic, overlying the tracheal cartilages.

D. Incorrect. Tracheal rings are illustrated by the *yellow arrow*.

Refer to the following figure for questions 8.5 to 8.7.

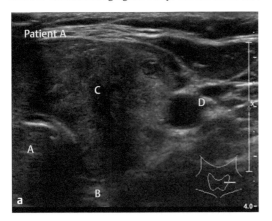

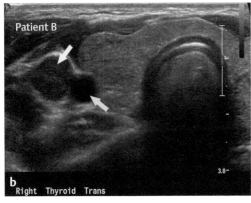

Question 8.5: Patient A is 57-year-old female who complains of voice changes. Neck ultrasound reveals enlargement of the left lobe of the thyroid gland. Compression at what point likely accounts for her symptoms?

A. A.

B. B.

C. C.

D. D.

Question 8.6: Patient B demonstrates a lesion (*yellow arrow*) that splays the internal jugular vein (IJV) (compressed) and the common carotid artery (*blue arrow*). From which structure does it likely arise?

A. Accessory spinal nerve.

B. Recurrent laryngeal nerve.

C. Vagus nerve.

D. Hypoglossal nerve.

Question 8.7: What underlying pathology best accounts for the finding in patient B?

A. Sturge–Weber syndrome.

B. Follicular thyroid cancer.

C. Neurofibromatosis.

D. Sarcoidosis.

Answer 8.5:

B. Correct. The recurrent laryngeal nerve (branch of the vagus nerve) runs in space between the trachea and medial aspect of the thyroid lobes. It provides motor supply to the vocal cords. Enlargement of the thyroid may result in compression of the recurrent laryngeal nerve, leading to hoarseness.

A. Incorrect. (A) represents the trachea.

C. Incorrect. (C) represents the substance of the enlarged left lobe of the thyroid.

D. Incorrect. (D) represents the carotid sheath containing the internal jugular vein, common carotid artery, and the vagus nerve.

Answer 8.6:

C. Correct. The vagus nerve runs within the carotid sheath along with the IJV and common carotid artery.

A. Incorrect. This not the anatomic location of the accessory spinal nerve.

B. Incorrect. This not the anatomic location of the recurrent laryngeal nerve.

D. Incorrect. This not the anatomic location of the hypoglossal nerve.

Answer 8.7:

C. Correct. Patient B is known to have neurofibromatosis type 2 with multiple nerve sheath tumors including the one in this case. The location of the lesion predicts its neural origin.

A. Incorrect. Sturge–Weber syndrome is characterized by port-wine stains involving the face and angiomas of the pia mater. There is an association with paragangliomas which technically include glomus vagale tumors. However, these typically occur at the common carotid bifurcation, splaying the internal and external carotid arteries. This rather tenuous link is, therefore, not the correct option.

B. Incorrect. Follicular thyroid cancer typically metastasizes via the hematogenous route. Hence regional lymphadenopathy is not the best choice. On the other hand, papillary thyroid cancer frequently metastasizes via the lymphatics.

D. Incorrect. Sarcoidosis is a systemic disease characterized by noncaseating granulomas. Nodal disease typically involves the bilateral hilar and paratracheal regions. While cervical lymphadenopathy is possible, this is not the typical site.

Refer to the following figure for questions 8.8 to 8.10.

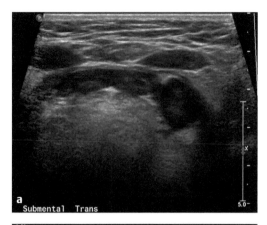

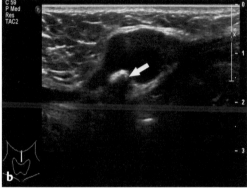

Question 8.8: This transverse submental view obtained from patient A demonstrates asymmetry. What is the likely diagnosis?
A. Thyroglossal duct cyst.
B. Lingual thyroid.
C. Metastatic disease.
D. Second branchial cleft cyst.

Question 8.9: This longitudinal midline view of the neck, at the level of the hyoid bone (*yellow arrow*), was obtained in patient B. This patient was suspected to have thyroid cancer recurrence based on a radioiodine scan. What explains this finding?
A. Lymphangioma.
B. Thyroglossal duct cyst.
C. Recurrent thyroid cancer.
D. Ranula.

Question 8.10: What maneuver may assist with the diagnosis in patient B?
A. Erect and supine posture.
B. Lateral decubitus positioning.
C. Tongue protrusion.
D. Valsalva.

Answer 8.8:
C. Correct. Patient A has biopsy-proven squamous cell carcinoma at the base of the tongue. The lesion with the left aspect of the floor of the mouth represents a metastatic deposit.

A. Incorrect. A thyroglossal duct cyst is a fluid-filled cavity occurring along the path of embryologic decent of the thyroid. It is typically midline in location and may contain ectopic thyroid tissue. This lesion typically elevates on tongue protrusion.

B. Incorrect. A lingual thyroid occurs typically when normal descent of the thyroid gland from the base of the tongue to the mid neck does not occur. Most often, the ectopic thyroid gland is entirely located at the base of the tongue, within the midline, with no thyroid tissue demonstrable within the usual pretracheal location. This image demonstrates a small, hypoechoic lesion far away from midline.

D. Incorrect. A second branchial cleft cyst is a developmental anomaly resulting in the formation of a cystic lesion which is typically located anterior to sternocleidomastoid muscle.

Answer 8.9:
B. Correct. Patient B demonstrates the classic appearance and location of a thyroglossal duct cyst. As already mentioned, a thyroglossal duct cyst is fluid-filled cavity occurring along the path of embryologic decent of the thyroid. It is typically midline in location and may contain ectopic thyroid tissue. This accounts for the activity seen on thyroid tissue sensitive nuclear medicine studies.

A. Incorrect. A lymphangioma is a benign fluid-filled lesion occurring typically around the head and neck in the pediatric population. They are also known as cystic hygromas and tend to contain septations.

C. Incorrect. Recurrent thyroid cancer does not typically manifest as a purely cystic lesion.

D. Incorrect. A ranula is a type of retention cyst usually occurring in the sublingual space, off midline, as a result of sublingual glandular infection or trauma.

Answer 8.10:
C. Correct. The attachment of the thyroglossal duct cyst to the base of the tongue results in elevation of the lesion on tongue protrusion.

A, B, D—Incorrect. These maneuvers would not be helpful.

Refer to the following figure for questions 8.11 to 8.13.

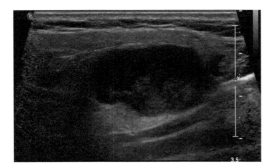

Question 8.11: This sonographic image of the left parotid gland of a 55-year-old chronic smoker demonstrates an abnormality. What is the most likely diagnosis?

A. Pleomorphic adenoma.
B. Warthin tumor.
C. Parotid cyst.
D. Hemangioma.

Question 8.12: The above lesion was biopsied. Which of the following clinical manifestations suggests nerve injury?

A. Ipsilateral face droop and forehead paralysis.
B. Contralateral face droop and forehead paralysis.
C. Contralateral face droop and preserved forehead motor function.
D. Ipsilateral face droop and preserved forehead motor function.

Question 8.13: A Tc-99m pertechnetate scan was undertaken for another unrelated indication. Incidental observations were made with regard to the parotid lesion. Which of the following is true?

A. A cold lesion excludes benignity.
B. A hot lesion is most often malignant.
C. A hot lesion is suggestive of Warthin tumor.
D. Tc-99m pertechnetate is useful in differentiating the different types of parotid malignancies.

Answer 8.11:

B. Correct. Warthin tumors are the second most common benign tumors of the parotid gland, be-hind pleomorphic adenomas. Warthin tumors are slow-growing and occur typically in middle-aged men with a history of smoking. They are hy-poechoic on ultrasound with occasional cystic spaces. Posterior acoustic enhancement may also be present. The appearance and location of the lesion, coupled with the history, make option B the correct choice.

A. Incorrect. Given the clinical context, option A is incorrect. However, pleomorphic adenomas may share some sonographic features with the Warthin tumor.

C. Incorrect. Parotid cysts are uncommon. When present, they are typically well-defined and an-echoic.

D. Incorrect. Parotid hemangiomas typically occur in the pediatric population. They may contain phle-boliths, typically seen as punctate echogenic foci.

Answer 8.12:

A. Correct. Facial nerve injury is uncommon during parotid fine needle aspiration (FNA). If injury or compression of the nerve ensues, say from a large intraparotid hematoma or subsequent abscess, this may manifest as a lower motor neuron type injury characterized by ipsilateral face droop and ipsilat-eral forehead paralysis. Recall, the facial nerve gives rise to five terminal branches within the parotid gland, which supply the muscles of facial expres-sion. Insults occurring proximal to the brainstem result in contralateral facial droop and preservation of forehead motor function due to cross-over/dual forehead innervation at this level.

B, C, D—Incorrect. These are not the signs of a lower motor neuron injury.

Answer 8.13:

C. Correct. Parotid malignancies manifest as cold lesion on Tc-99m pertechnetate studies. Pleomor-phic adenomas are also "cold" on this study which helps to differentiate them from a Warthin tumor which is typically hot due to an abundance of mito-chondria within oncocytes.

A, B, D—Incorrect. These options are incorrect due to the above mentioned reason.

Refer to the following figure for questions 8.14 to 8.16.

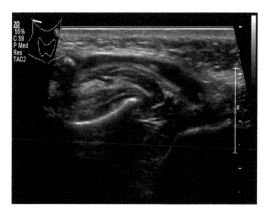

Question 8.14: This transverse image of the right cheek, taken at the level of the upper maxilla demonstrates what pathology?
A. Sialolithiasis.
B. Thrombophlebitis.
C. Cellulitis.
D. Sialadenitis.

Question 8.15: This pathology is encountered most frequently in which location?
A. Parotid glands.
B. Sublingual glands.
C. Submandibular gland.
D. Accessory salivary glands.

Question 8.16: What is the term for sialadenitis due to ductal obstruction from a mucus plug?
A. Kussmaul disease.
B. Kuttner's tumor.
C. Kimura's disease.
D. Mikulicz's disease.

Answer 8.14:
A. Correct. The image demonstrates distention of the main duct of the parotid gland, also known as Stensen's duct. With the duct there are several calculi, the largest of which sits just inferior to the body maker at the upper left corner of the image. Sialolithiasis is the second most common cause of sialadenitis next only to mumps.

B. Incorrect. The imaged tubular structure is the main parotid duct, not a vein.

C. Incorrect. There are no imaging features to support this diagnosis.

D. Incorrect. The actual parotid gland is not imaged. Hence, a diagnosis of sialadenitis cannot be made on the basis of this image.

Answer 8.15:
C. Correct. Sialolithiasis is very common in the submandibular gland and may cause diffuse or focal enlargement of the gland. Thick, alkaline saliva coupled with the uphill course of Wharton's duct (main duct of the submandibular gland) may account for this observation.

A, B, D—Incorrect. Sialolithiasis most frequently affects the submandibular gland.

Answer 8.16:
A. Correct. Kussmaul disease (sialodochitis fibrinosa) is described as an acute episode of sialadenitis secondary to obstruction of the main duct.

B. Incorrect. A "Kuttner's tumor" describes a palpable firm, mass-like submandibular gland due to chronic inflammation.

C. Incorrect. Kimura's disease is a chronic inflammatory disease of the cervical lymph nodes and salivary glands. It is characterized by eosinophilia and markedly elevated serum IgE. It typically afflicts Asian males.

D. Incorrect. Mikulicz's syndrome is a variant of Sjogren's syndrome characterized by inflammation of two or more salivary and lacrimal glands. Xerostomia is also present.

Question 8.17: The cystic lesions of the parotid gland shown below in patient A are most commonly encountered with which pathogen?

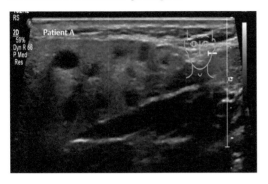

A. Cytomegalovirus.
B. Human immunodeficiency virus (HIV).
C. Hepatitis B virus.
D. Mycobacterium tuberculosis.

Answer:
B. Correct. Patient A demonstrates multiple cystic lesions throughout the parotid gland. These findings are typical of benign lymphoepithelial lesions, a frequent finding in patients with HIV infection. The parotid glands are most frequently affected and there is an association with cervical lymph node enlargement.

A. Incorrect. Cytomegalovirus is not associated with parotid cysts.

C. Incorrect. Hepatitis B virus is not associated with parotid cysts.

D. Incorrect. Mycobacterium tuberculosis is not associated with parotid cysts.

Question 8.18: Patient B is a 31-year-old female. A sonographic image of one of her parotid glands is presented. Which of the following is true?

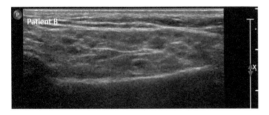

A. The findings are consistent with Sjogren's disease.
B. The findings are within normal limits.
C. This appearance should prompt a thorough search for intraparotid lymph nodes, since lymph nodes in the parotid gland are usually abnormal.
D. None of the above.

Answer:
A. Correct. This image was obtained from an adult female patient with Sjogren's disease. The typical sonographic appearance includes multiple hypoechoic foci throughout the gland correlating with aggregates of lymphocytes.

B. Incorrect. The normal parotid gland typically demonstrates smooth echotexture and is homogenously echogenic.

C. Incorrect. While there is an increased risk of developing Non-Hodgkin's lymphoma in patients with Sjogren's disease, intraparotid lymph nodes are normal findings. Late embryologic encapsulation results in normal lymph nodes being incorporated within the parotid.

D. Incorrect.

Question 8.19: In this sonographic image, which structure is represented by the *yellow arrow*?

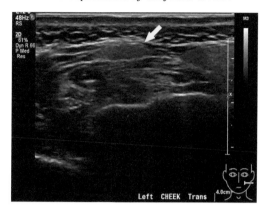

A. An abnormal lymph node.
B. A normal variant.
C. A normal lymph node.
D. None of the above.

Answer:
B. Correct. The *arrow* indicates an accessory parotid gland, a normal variant. Typically, the accessory gland is located anterior to the main parotid gland and derives its separate blood supply from the transverse facial artery. It drains via a separate duct to the main parotid duct. Any pathology affecting the parotid glands can also affect the accessory parotid.

A. Incorrect. This accessory parotid gland demonstrates a smooth, homogenously echogenic appearance, identical to the main parotid gland. This would be an unusual appearance for a lymph node, normal or abnormal.

C. Incorrect. A normal lymph node is typically reniform and demonstrates an echogenic hilum. These findings are not present.

D. Incorrect.

Question 8.20: Based on the images below, what likely accounts for the abnormal appearance of the submandibular glands of this 35-year-old male patient?

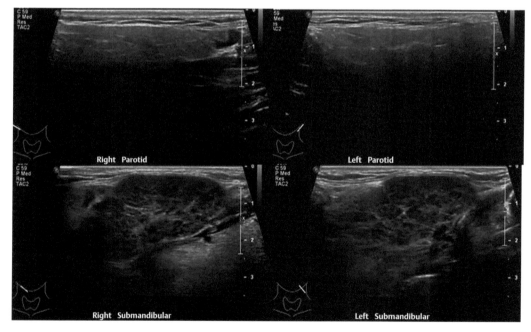

A. Therapeutic radioiodine changes 5 years after treatment.
B. Sjogren's disease.
C. Parvovirus infection.
D. Sarcoidosis.

Answer:
D. Correct. The images demonstrate normal parotid glands and with enlarged, heterogeneously hypoechoic submandibular glands. Sarcoidosis may involve both the parotid and submandibular

glands. However, sole submandibular gland involvement is more frequent than sole parotid involvement.

A. Incorrect. The submandibular glands are frequently affected by radiotherapy-induced changes secondary to thyroid malignancy treatment. However, after a few years, the glands are usually relatively atrophic and small as opposed to enlarged as seen in this case.

B. Incorrect. Sjogren's syndrome is a chronic autoimmune disorder affecting the lacrimal and salivary glands. Patients typically demonstrate, dry eyes, dry mouth, and bilateral parotid swelling. On ultrasound the parotid glands are noted be enlarged with varying echogenicity, hyperechoic in the early stages and hypoechoic/multicystic later on in the disease course.

C. Incorrect. Parvovirus infection (mumps) typically affects the parotid gland.

Refer to the following figure for questions 8.21 and 8.22.

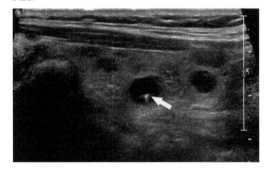

Question 8.21: This longitudinal sonographic view of the left lobe of the thyroid demonstrates a rounded thyroid lesion. Which option is consistent with appropriate management?
A. FNA.
B. Thorough neck ultrasound to exclude a primary malignancy.
C. Antibiotics.
D. No further action required.

Question 8.22: What type of artifact is demonstrated by the *yellow arrow* in the image?
A. Reverberation.
B. Mirror image.
C. Shadowing.
D. Side lobe.

Answer 8.21:
D. Correct. The image demonstrates a well-defined almost purely cystic lesion with a contained echogenic focus demonstrating a "comet tail." This is the classic appearance of a colloid cyst, a benign entity requiring no further management.

A. Incorrect. Colloid cysts are benign and do not require FNA.

B. Incorrect. Colloid cysts are benign. They are not associated with malignancies.

C. Incorrect. Antibiotics would be inappropriate as there is no underlying infection.

Answer 8.22:
A. Correct. The *arrow* indicates an echogenic focus with an associated "comet tail," commonly referred to as comet tail artifact. This is a type of reverberation artifact caused by sound "bouncing" back and forth between two closely spaced reflective surfaces. Pure reverberation artifact results in a repetitive display of equally spaced echogenic lines. However, for comet tail artifact, the echogenic lines are so close together that they are perceived as one entity. The later (and hence deeper) echoes are more attenuated and thus are displayed with diminished widths, leading to the tapered or triangular appearance.

B. Incorrect. Mirror image artifact is also due to multiple reflections of the primary ultrasound beam usually from a highly reflective surface deep to the duplicated structure. The mirror image is displayed at an equal distance on the opposite side of the reflector.

C. Incorrect. Shadowing occurs when transmission of sound through a structure is poor relative to the adjacent structures resulting in a dark band or "shadow" deep to the imaged structure.

D. Incorrect. Side lobes are weak off-axis ultrasound beams. If they encounter a very strong reflector which is lateral to the main scan line, the reflector may be erroneously placed within the path of the main scan line. This artifact is more obvious when an anechoic structure occupies the main scan line, such as a full urinary bladder.

Refer to the following figure for questions 8.23 to 8.25.

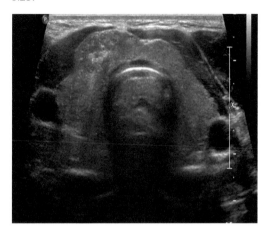

Question 8.23: What unique entity does this ill-defined lesion within the right lobe of the thyroid likely contain?
A. Koilocytes.
B. Parafollicular C cells.
C. Hurthle cells.
D. Psammoma bodies.

Question 8.24: In general, what sonographic feature is felt to predict malignancy in thyroid nodules?
A. Wider than tall.
B. Very hyperechoic.
C. Ill-defined margins.
D. Solid composition.

Question 8.25: The above lesion was biopsied. Which specimen is deemed adequate?
A. Little to no blood within the specimen and four follicular groups.
B. At least six follicular groups.
C. At least five follicular groups and the absence of ultrasound gel within the specimen.
D. Scant colloid and at least four follicular groups.

Answer 8.23:
D. Correct. Psammoma bodies are tiny areas of lamellated calcification. These are frequently encountered in papillary carcinoma of the thyroid and manifest as multiple tiny echogenic foci.

A. Incorrect. Koilocytes are associated with human papillomavirus infection.

B. Incorrect. Parafollicular C cells are the site of origin of medullary thyroid cancer.

C. Incorrect. Hurthle cells are typically associated with Hashimoto's thyroiditis or a variant of follicular thyroid carcinoma.

Answer 8.24:
D. Correct. The relatively new thyroid imaging reporting and data system (TIRADS) classification scores thyroid nodules with respect to composition, margin, echogenicity, shape, and echogenic foci. The points allocated for each category are summated and the higher the score, the greater the likelihood of malignancy. A solid or predominately solid nodule scores 2 points, the highest for the "composition category."

A. Incorrect. A taller than wide nodule is more suspicious than vice versa and scores maximum (3 points) for the "shape" category.

B. Incorrect. A very hypoechoic nodule scores the maximum of 3 points for the "echogenicity" category.

C. Incorrect. Though somewhat counterintuitive, a nodule with ill-defined margins actually scores zero for the "margin" category. A lobulated or irregular margin scores 2 points whereas extrathyroid extension scores 3.

Answer 8.25:
B. Correct. A thyroid nodule FNA sample is deemed adequate if there are 6 well-preserved groups of follicular cells, each containing at least 10 cells.

A, C, D—Incorrect. These are not deemed adequate.

Refer to the following figure for questions 8.26 to 8.28.

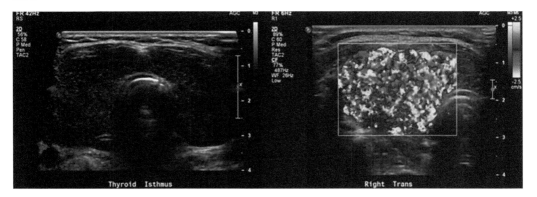

Question 8.26: Sonographic images of the thyroid gland are shown above. What is the most likely diagnosis?

A. Graves' disease.

B. Hashimoto's thyroiditis.

C. Lymphoma.

D. Thyroid abscess.

Question 8.27: What further abnormality is probably present?

A. Antithyroglobulin antibodies.

B. Elevated T3 and T4.

C. Neck pain and preceding history of a viral infection.

D. IgG4-related sclerosing disease.

Question 8.28: Which of the following is employed in the diagnosis of this disease?

A. ^{123}I-NaI.

B. ^{123}I-meta-iodobenzylguanidine (^{123}I-MIBG).

C. ^{123}I-DaTscan.

D. None of the above.

Answer 8.26:
A. Correct. Graves' disease is an autoimmune disease affecting the thyroid gland caused by antibodies that target thyroid-stimulating hormone (TSH) receptors. On ultrasound, the gland is swollen and diffusely hypoechoic. Color Doppler demonstrates markedly increased vascularity described as "thyroid inferno." These features are demonstrated in the provided images.

B. Incorrect. Hashimoto's thyroiditis is typically characterized by an enlarged hypoechoic gland with heterogeneous echotexture with bright fibrotic bands. Vascularity on color Doppler is variable and, while thyroid inferno may rarely occur, it is more likely to be associated with Graves' disease.

C. Incorrect. Thyroid lymphoma typically presents as a heterogeneously enlarged thyroid without normal intervening parenchyma. Extracapsular extension may also be present. The most common type of thyroid lymphoma is mucosa-associated lymphoid tissue lymphoma, followed by diffuse large B-cell lymphoma. Patients may present with obstructive symptoms due to compression of the airways.

D. Incorrect. A thyroid abscess is an infrequent complication of thyroiditis or other neck inflammatory process. Like abscesses elsewhere in the body, it is characterized by a hypoechoic fluid collection with peripheral hyperemia.

Answer 8.27:
B. Correct. Graves' thyroiditis is an autoimmune disorder characterized by thyrotoxicosis with an observed increase in both T3 and T4 levels. TSH levels are suppressed.

A. Incorrect. Antithyroglobulin antibodies are typically encountered in Hashimoto's thyroiditis.

C. Incorrect. Neck pain and preceding history of a viral infection are associated with De Quervain's thyroiditis.

D. Incorrect. IgG4-related sclerosing disease is associated with Riedel's thyroiditis. Examples of IgG4-related sclerosing disease include autoimmune pancreatitis and sclerosing mesenteritis.

Answer 8.28:
A. Correct. ^{123}I-NaI scan and uptake are the standard exams to assess patients with Graves' disease. ^{123}I-NaI has a half-life of 13.22 hours and emits gamma radiation with a 159-keV energy peak, which is suitable for medical imaging. It also allows for uptake measurements which is used for subsequent therapeutic dosage determination.

B. Incorrect. ^{123}I-MIBG is a norepinephrine analogue that is used for the assessment and staging of patents with neuroblastoma and pheochromocytoma but not Grave's disease, although labelled with [123]I.

C. Incorrect. ^{123}I-DaTscan is a cocaine analogue with high affinity to dopamine transporter (DaT) located on the presynaptic nerve endings in the striatum. It is clinically used to differentiate essential tremor from Parkinsonian syndromes. It is also one of the ^{123}I-labelled radiopharmaceuticals that is not used for assessment of Grave's disease.

D. Incorrect. ^{123}I-NaI is useful in the work-up of patients with Graves' disease.

Refer to the following figure for questions 8.29 and 8.30.

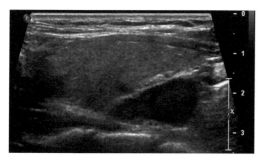

Question 8.29: Sagittal view of the right lobe of the thyroid gland in a patient with neck fullness. What additional clinical symptom(s) may be present?

A. Dysphagia.
B. Heat intolerance.
C. Rigors and malaise.
D. Constipation.

Question 8.30: What recommendation should be made to the referring clinician as the logical next step in management of the patient?

A. Positron emission tomography/computed tomography (PET/CT) from head to mid-thigh to evaluate for primary malignancy.
B. FNA.
C. Serum biochemical analysis.
D. Course of antibiotics.

Answer 8.29:
D. Correct. The ultrasound image demonstrates a well-defined hypoechoic structure along the posterior surface of the thyroid gland. This is the classic appearance of a parathyroid adenoma. The ensuing hyperparathyroidism leads to hypercalcemia and the classic "stones, painful bones, psychic moans and intestinal groans" (hypercalcemia-induced constipation).

A. Incorrect. Dysphagia may be associated with a goitrous enlargement of the thyroid.

B. Incorrect. Heat intolerance is associated with hyperthyroidism.

C. Incorrect. Rigors and malaise suggest underlying infection.

Answer 8.30:
C. Correct. Parathyroid hormone levels and serum calcium may be increased.

A. Incorrect. PET/CT would be inappropriate as there is no underlying malignancy.

B. Incorrect. FNA of a parathyroid adenoma can be helpful by determining the presence of parathormone (PTH) within the aspirate. However, parathyroid FNA can lead to extensive fibrosis, thus rendering surgical excision challenging. Also, the associated fibrosis may be confused with malignancy at histology. Consequently, FNA of parathyroid adenomas is typically avoided in some centers.

D. Incorrect. A course of antibiotic would be inappropriate.

Refer to the following figure for questions 8.31 and 8.32.

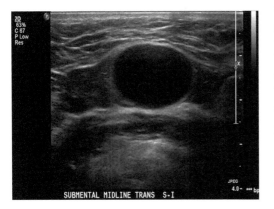

Question 8.31: You are reviewing this image of a midline transverse view of the submental region with the ultrasound technologist. The patient is in the scanning room. What should be the next step in imaging?

A. FNA after contacting the referring service.

B. No further imaging/workup is required as the finding is clearly benign.

C. A contrast-enhanced CT of the neck is highly recommended while the patient is still within the radiology department.

D. None of the above.

Question 8.32: At what level in the neck is the lesion?

A. Level 1.

B. Level 2.

C. Level 3.

D. Level 4.

Answer 8.31:

D. Correct. This submental nodule is rounded and very hypoechoic. Though it may appear cystic, the lesion actually demonstrated internal vascular flow on color Doppler imaging. Therefore, the next step should be to further evaluate with color Doppler.

A. Incorrect. After evaluating with Doppler, FNA would be appropriate.

B. Incorrect. The lesion was eventually biopsied and confirmed to be lymphoma.

C. Incorrect. A CT of the neck may be appropriate later on in the workup.

Answer 8.32:

A. Correct. Head and neck surgeons as well as pathologists use a simplified numeric classification system to reproducibly identify the locations of cervical lymph nodes. Level 1 lymph nodes are located beneath the chin within the submental or submandibular regions. Quite often, a lymph node is located between the anterior bellies of the digastric muscles, as is the case in this patient with lymphoma.

B. Incorrect. A level 2 lymph node is situated within the internal jugular/deep cervical chain from the level of the skull base to the inferior border of the hyoid bone.

C. Incorrect. A level 3 lymph node is situated within the internal jugular/deep cervical chain from the level of the hyoid bone to the cricoid.

D. Incorrect. A level 4 lymph node is situated within the internal jugular/deep cervical chain from the level of the cricoid to the supraclavicular fossa.

Further Readings

Ahuja A, Evans R, eds. Practical Head and Neck Ultrasound. Cambridge: Cambridge University Press; 2000

Ahuja AT. Diagnostic Imaging Ultrasound. Salt Lake City: Amirysis; 2007

Anderson L, Middleton WD, Teefey SA, et al. Hashimoto thyroiditis: part 1, sonographic analysis of the nodular form of Hashimoto thyroiditis. AJR Am J Roentgenol 2010;195(1):208–215

Bialek EJ, Jakubowski W, Zajkowski P, Szopinski KT, Osmolski A. US of the major salivary glands: anatomy and spatial relationships, pathologic conditions, and pitfalls. Radiographics 2006;26(3):745–763

Bravo E, Grayev A. Thyroid abscess as a complication of bacterial throat infection. J Radiol Case Rep 2011;5(3):1–7

Chong V. Cervical lymphadenopathy: what radiologists need to know. Cancer Imaging 2004; 4(2):116–120

Dähnert W. Radiology Review Manual. Philadelphia, PA: Wolters Kluwer; 2011

Feldman MK, Katyal S, Blackwood MS. US artifacts. Radiographics 2009;29(4):1179–1189

Goellner JR, Gharib H, Grant CS, Johnson DA. Fine needle aspiration cytology of the thyroid, 1980 to 1986. Acta Cytol 1987;31(5):587–590

Grant EG, Tessler FN, Hoang JK, et al. Thyroid Ultrasound Reporting Lexicon: White Paper of the ACR Thyroid Imaging, Reporting and Data System (TIRADS) Committee. J Am Coll Radiol 2015;12(12 Pt A):1272–1279

Martinoli C, Pretolesi F, Del Bono V, Derchi LE, Mecca D, Chiaramondia M. Benign lymphoepithelial parotid lesions in HIV-positive patients: spectrum of findings at gray-scale and Doppler sonography. AJR Am J Roentgenol 1995;165(4):975–979

Nachiappan AC, Metwalli ZA, Hailey BS, Patel RA, Ostrowski ML, Wynne DM. The thyroid: review of imaging features and biopsy techniques with radiologic-pathologic correlation. Radiographics 2014;34(2):276–293

Netter FH. Atlas of Human Anatomy. Philadelphia, PA: Saunders/Elsevier; 2011

Norman J, Politz D, Browarsky I. Diagnostic aspiration of parathyroid adenomas causes severe fibrosis complicating surgery and final histologic diagnosis. Thyroid 2007;17(12):1251–1255

Oh J-R, Ahn B-C. False-positive uptake on radioiodine whole-body scintigraphy: physiologic and pathologic variants unrelated to thyroid cancer. Am J Nucl Med Mol Imaging 2012;2(3):362–385

Ramachar SM, Huliyappa HA. Accessory parotid gland tumors. Ann Maxillofac Surg 2012;2(1):90–93

Rastogi R, Bhargava S, Mallarajapatna GJ, Singh SK. Pictorial essay: salivary gland imaging. Indian J Radiol Imaging 2012;22(4):325–333

Yamamoto M, Harada S, Ohara M, et al. Clinical and pathological differences between Mikulicz's disease and Sjögren's syndrome. Rheumatology (Oxford) 2005; 44(2):227–234

Yousem DM, Kraut MA, Chalian AA. Major salivary gland imaging. Radiology 2000;216(1):19–29

Zander DA, Smoker WR. Imaging of ectopic thyroid tissue and thyroglossal duct cysts. Radiographics 2014; 34(1):37–50

Chapter 9

Scrotum

Barbara Pawley and Adrian Dawkins

9 Questions and Answers

Question 9.1: In the transverse view of the testis, what does the *yellow arrow* indicate?

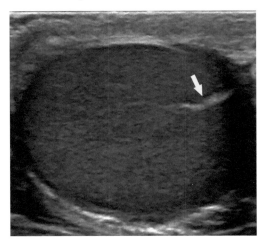

A. Convergence of the seminiferous tubules.
B. Reverberation artifact.
C. Focal scarring from prior infection.
D. Tunica vaginalis.

Answer:

A. Correct. The *yellow arrow* indicates the mediastinum testis, representing the point at which the seminiferous tubules converge.

B. Incorrect. Reverberation artifact is seen as a series of equally spaced parallel lines due to multiple reflections of sound between two closely spaced structures.

C. Incorrect. The mediastinum testis is a normal anatomic structure and not the result of scarring.

D. Incorrect. The tunica vaginalis is not invested into the parenchyma of the testis.

Question 9.2: Which of the following statements is correct? The tunica vaginalis_____.
A. Is a single layer.
B. Is deep to the tunica albuginea.
C. Is a mesothelium-lined sac.
D. None of the above.

Answer:

C. Correct. The tunica vaginalis is a mesothelium-lined sac. Consequently, lesions of mesothelial origin may occur, manifesting as extratesticular masses. Such lesions include adenomatoid tumor and mesothelioma.

A. Incorrect. The tunica vaginalis forms two layers, the parietal and visceral layers. These are splayed in the setting of a hydrocele.

B. Incorrect. The layers of the tunica vaginalis are superficial to the tunica albuginea. The tunica albuginea is a fibrous layer that closely invests the testis.

D. Incorrect.

Question 9.3: This patient was evaluated for a possible inguinal hernia. The *yellow arrowhead* indicates the right epididymis. The left epididymis demonstrated a similar appearance. What is the most likely explanation?

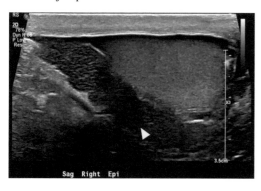

A. Epididymitis.
B. Torsion.
C. Right renal mass.
D. Vasectomy.

Answer:

D. Correct. The epididymis in enlarged and demonstrates a speckled appearance. This has been described as tubular ectasia of the epididymis and is a frequent finding in patients who have undergone a vasectomy.

A. Incorrect. There is no supportive evidence to suggest acute inflammation of the testis and/or epididymis as there is no demonstrated hypervascularity.

B. Incorrect. There is no supportive evidence to suggest testicular torsion.

C. Incorrect. A right renal mass, with venous invasion, may lead to a right varicocele due to obstruction of the right testicular vein. However, a varicocele was not imaged.

Question 9.4: A patient with a prior history of a vasectomy presents with a lump within the right hemiscrotum, superior to and separate from the testis. What is the likely diagnosis?

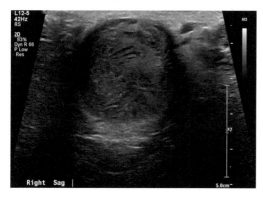

A. Abscess.
B. Epidermoid cyst.
C. Adenomatoid tumor.
D. Sperm cell granuloma.

Answer:

D. Correct. The image demonstrates a solid rounded well-defined mass. While the imaging appearances are somewhat nonspecific, the history of a prior vasectomy coupled with the location make a sperm cell granuloma the likely diagnosis. A sperm cell granuloma forms from chronic inflammation in response to a prior vasectomy and tends to occur with the epididymis or along the vasa deferentia.

A. Incorrect. An abscess presents as a complex fluid collection with surround hypervascularity.

B. Incorrect. An epidermoid cyst is typically an intratesticular lesion.

C. Incorrect. An adenomatoid tumor is the most common extratesticular tumor and is typically solid and well defined. It is certainly a worthy differential consideration for this finding, however the history of a prior vasectomy renders this a less likely choice.

Question 9.5: This patient was evaluated for a scrotal mass. The tubular structure being measured was confirmed to be a vessel with Doppler imaging. Which statement is correct?

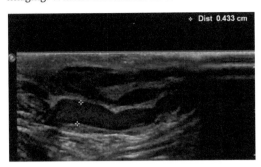

A. This finding is more frequent on the right.

B. The caliber of the vessel is within normal limits.

C. Apparent echogenic material within the vessel is due to thrombus.

D. The finding may result in subfertility.

Answer:

D. Correct. The image demonstrates dilated vessels within the hemiscrotum. This is the classic appearance of a varicocele, dilation of the pampiniform venous plexus above 3 mm. This typically results from reversal of flow within the testicular vein and is much more common on the left, presumably due to the horizontal course of the left renal vein, into which the left testicular vein drains. The Valsalva maneuver results in an exacerbation of the findings due to reflux. Patients with varicoceles may develop subfertility due to impaired spermatogenesis in part due to the increased local temperature caused by dilated veins.

A, B—Incorrect. Refer to the explanation of the correct choice above.

C. Incorrect. The apparent echogenic material within the vein is artifactual secondary to slow flow.

Question 9.6: A 10-year-old boy presents with left testicular pain. A scrotal ultrasound is obtained, an image from which is demonstrated below. What is the likely diagnosis?

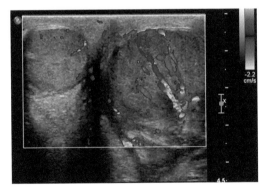

A. Orchitis.

B. Epididymitis.

C. Left testicular torsion.

D. Germ cell tumor.

Answer:

A. Correct. The image demonstrates a swollen left testis with increase vascular flow, the typical appearance of acute orchitis.

B. Incorrect. While epididymitis frequently occurs in conjunction with orchitis, the left epididymis is not imaged. Therefore, epididymitis cannot be confirmed on the current images.

C. Incorrect. Decreased vascular flow is expected within the affected testes in cases of acute torsion.

D. Incorrect. A discrete testicular mass is not imaged.

Question 9.7: After 2 weeks of treatment, a patient with acute orchitis returns for a follow-up ultrasound. Which statement best describes this new appearance?

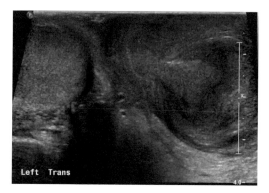

A. There has been inadequate treatment of underlying infection.
B. The testis is now devitalized secondary to progression of intermittent torsion.
C. An enlarging hematoma is present.
D. There has been progression of aggressive neoplasm.

Answer:
A. Correct. The image demonstrates suppurative material exuding from the left testes, beyond the tunica albuginea. The findings are consistent with rupture of an intratesticular abscess, leading to a pyocele. This occurred secondary to inadequate antibiotic treatment of orchitis.

B. Incorrect. Established torsion would manifest as heterogeneity of the testicular parenchyma and an absence of vascular flow.

C. Incorrect. A hematoma is not present.

D. Incorrect. An underlying neoplasm is not present.

Question 9.8: A 28-year-old male presents with a painless testicular lump. A scrotal ultrasound was performed, an image from which is presented here. Which statement is correct?

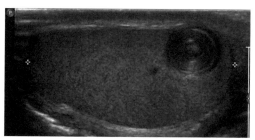

A. This finding is most frequently associated with microlithiasis.
B. This lesion is almost certainly benign.
C. An orchiectomy is the most appropriate treatment.
D. A course of antibiotics would be appropriate.

Answer:
B. Correct. The image demonstrates a well-defined, rounded intratesticular lesion within a lamellated or "onion-skin" appearance. These finding are typical of an epidermoid cyst, a benign lesion.

A. Incorrect. The epidermoid cyst is not associated with microlithiasis.

C. Incorrect. This lesion may be enucleated, sparing the testis.

D. Incorrect. A course of antibiotics is not indicated.

Question 9.9: An 18-year-old male straddles a wooden fence. He presents 2 weeks later with scrotal swelling and undergoes an ultrasound. The testes are normal. Given the finding below, what management strategy is appropriate?

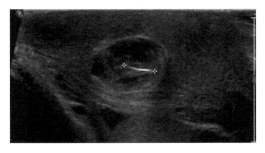

A. Administration of antibiotics.
B. Obtain a pelvic radiograph.
C. Local incision.
D. None of the above.

Answer:
C. Correct. The image demonstrates a slender echogenic line within a surrounding well-defined hypoechoic focus situated within the edematous scrotal skin. This finding is consistent with a retained wooden splinter with a surrounding "foreign body granuloma." A local incision, especially if guided by sonographic marking, would facilitate retrieval.

A. Incorrect. Antibiotics would not provide definitive treatment for this condition.

B. Incorrect. A pelvic radiograph is unnecessary especially since wooden foreign bodies are often radiolucent.

D. Incorrect.

Question 9.10: A diabetic patient presents with groin pain and undergoes a scrotal ultrasound. Which statement is true regarding the finding below?

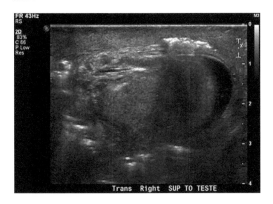

A. The scrotal skin demonstrates coarse calcification.
B. A retained foreign body is present.
C. Steroid administration is required.
D. None of the above.

Answer:
D. Correct. The image demonstrates gas within thickened scrotal skin, the hallmark of Fournier's gangrene. This life-threatening condition is most prevalent in middle-aged males, with diabetes being a predisposing factor. Urgent debridement and broad-spectrum antibiotics are required for an optimal outcome.

A. Incorrect. The echogenic foci within the scrotal skin demonstrate the classic "dirty shadowing" consistent with gas as opposed to calcification.

B. Incorrect. A retained foreign body is not imaged.

C. Incorrect. Steroids are not indicated.

Question 9.11: These sonographic images were obtained in a 46-year-old male with testicular pain. Of the options below, which best accounts for the findings?

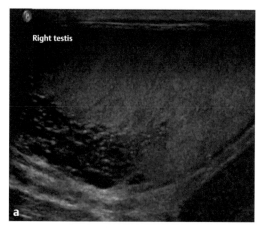

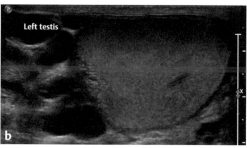

A. Ectasia of the rete testis and left spermatoceles.
B. Ectasia of the rete testis and left complex hydrocele.
C. Intratesticular varicocele and left spermatoceles.
D. Intratesticular varicocele and left complex hydrocele.

Answer:

A. Correct. The images demonstrate tubular cystic areas along the mediastinum testis, consistent with tubular ectasia of the rete testes. This is typically observed in middle-aged men and felt to be secondary to obstruction of the vasa efferentia, (the communicating tubular network between the rete testis and epididymal head). The condition is often bilateral though asymmetric. In the case presented, it is more marked on the right. Tubular ectasia of the rete testis is frequently associated with spermatoceles, a type of extratesticular cyst. Several spermatoceles are noted along the left testis.

B. Incorrect. A hydrocele occurs within the tunical space and typically surrounds the testis.

C. Incorrect. An intratesticular varicocele may create an appearance similar to tubular ectasia. However, the presence of vascular flow on Doppler imaging within an intratesticular varicocele and the classic location of tubular ectasia allow sonographic differentiation of these two entities.

D. Incorrect. A varicocele and hydrocele are not present.

Question 9.12 A 62-year-old male presents with testicular pain and undergoes a testicular ultrasound. Representative images are presented below. What is the most likely diagnosis?

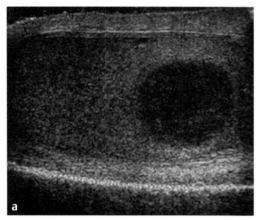

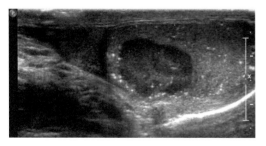

A. Seminoma.

B. Embryonal tumor.

C. Hematoma.

D. Lymphoma.

Answer:

D. Correct. The images demonstrate a well-defined hypoechoic mass with the testis. The mass is also avidly hypervascular. These findings, coupled with the patient's age, make lymphoma the most likely diagnosis. Testicular lymphoma is most often of the B cell variety.

A. Incorrect. Seminomas are the most common testicular tumor but typically occur in a younger demographic (average age of 40 years).

B. Incorrect. The sonographic features of this tumor are nonspecific but again, embryonal testicular tumor tends to occur in younger patients (25–35 years).

C. Incorrect. A hematoma is unlikely to show internal vascular flow.

Question 9.13: Regarding the image below which statement is correct?

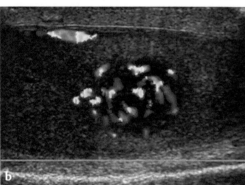

A. The lesion is most likely a Sertoli cell tumor.

B. The ipsilateral groin should be evaluated to excluded lymphatic spread since this is the first site of nodal disease.

C. Both of the above.

D. None of the above.

Answer:

D. Correct. The image demonstrates multiple tiny punctate echogenic foci throughout the testicular parenchyma, consistent with testicular microlithiasis. Testicular microlithiasis has been associated with the development of testicular tumors, in particular germ cell tumors such as seminomas. Testicular tumors first metastasize to paracaval lymph nodes consistent with lymphatic drainage.

A, B—Incorrect. Testicular tumors first metastasize to paracaval lymph nodes consistent with lymphatic drainage.

C. Incorrect.

Question 9.14: The image in (Question 9.13) demonstrates multiple tiny punctate echogenic foci throughout the testicular parenchyma, consistent with testicular microlithiasis. All the following are associated with the condition except?

A. Klinefelter syndrome.
B. Trisomy 21.
C. Alveolar proteinosis.
D. Klippel–Trenaunay syndrome.

Answer:

D. Correct. Klippel-Trenaunay syndrome is not associated with testicular microlithiasis.

A. Incorrect. Klinefelter syndrome is associated with testicular microlithiasis.

B. Incorrect. Trisomy 21 is associated with testicular microlithiasis.

C. Incorrect. Alveolar proteinosis is associated with testicular microlithiasis.

Question 9.15: A 26-year-old male presents with groin pain for which he undergoes a scrotal ultrasound. A representative image is demonstrated below. How should this finding be managed?

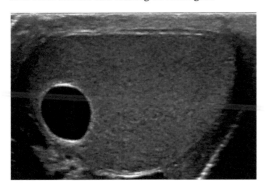

A. Orchiectomy.
B. Incision and drainage.
C. No intervention is necessary.
D. None of the above.

Answer:

C. Correct. The image demonstrates a well-defined anechoic intraparenchymal testicular cyst. These incidentally discovered lesions have no malignant potential and warrant no intervention.

A, B—Incorrect. No intervention is required.

D. Incorrect.

Question 9.16: A 17-year-old male presents with left testicular pain. He undergoes a scrotal ultrasound. Based on the images below, which statement is correct?

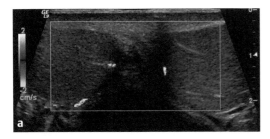

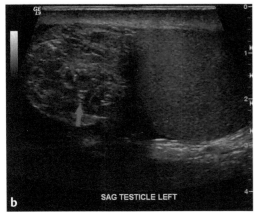

A. There is fairly symmetric vascular flow on color Doppler, effectively excluding testicular torsion.

B. The heterogenous mass at the upper aspect of the left testis is unlikely to represent a malignancy.

C. Both statements are correct.

D. Neither of the statements is correct.

Answer:

B. Correct. Intrascrotal, extratesticular masses are typically benign. The *red arrow* indicates a mass-like lesion at the superior aspect of the left testis. This demonstrates tubular internal contents and actually represents a "torsed" spermatic cord. It is to be remembered that testicular torsion is not actually twisting of the testis but rather twisting of the spermatic cord. For this reason, on clinical evaluation, the testis is not only tender, but also somewhat high-riding and more horizontal in lie. Consequently, the "exclude torsion" scanning protocol should always include an evaluation of the spermatic cord.

A. Incorrect. The subjective assessment of symmetric vascular flow is not sufficient to exclude testicular torsion. Instead, the absent or markedly decreased vascular flow within one testis may help support the diagnosis of torsion.

C, D—Incorrect.

Question 9.17: A 21-year-old patient presents with a roughly 2-week history of on and off scrotal pain. A scrotal ultrasound is performed. The images are consistent with which of the following conditions?

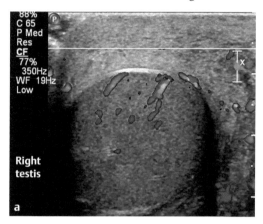

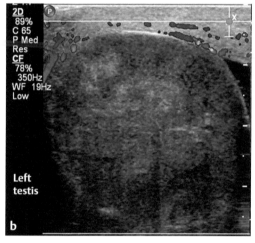

A. Right orchitis.
B. Left testicular neoplasm.
C. Left testicular infarction.
D. None of the above.

Answer:

C. Correct. The image demonstrates thickening of the scrotal skin and absent vascular flow within the heterogenous left testis. The findings are consistent with an infarcted left testis, secondary to torsion.

A. Incorrect. The vascular flow and parenchymal pattern of the right testis are within normal limits. There is typically increased vascular flow in the setting of orchitis.

B. Incorrect. Though there is heterogeneity throughout the left testicular parenchyma, a discrete mass in not identified making an underlying neoplasm unlikely.

D. Incorrect.

Question 9.18: A 21-year-old male presents with right groin pain. A scrotal ultrasound is performed. Based on the images below, which statement is correct?

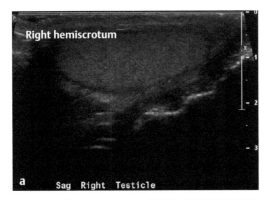

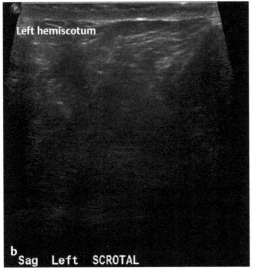

A. The right testis is normal but the left testis is likely to be congenitally absent.

B. The right testis is normal. An inguinal hernia is probably obscuring the left testis.

C. Both kidneys should be evaluated since there is a high likelihood of associated renal agenesis.

D. The ipsilateral groin and spermatic cord should be sonographically evaluated.

Answer:

D. Correct. In the setting of an incidentally discovered "absent testis," an undescended testis/cryptorchidism should be excluded. Usually, the undescended testis is located within the ipsilateral groin and hence frequently amenable to sonographic visualization.

A. Incorrect. Undescended testis is much more likely than congenital absence of the testis.

B. Incorrect. In the setting of an intrascrotal inguinal hernia, the testis is still usually visible, albeit often displaced inferiorly within the scrotum.

C. Incorrect. There is no strong correlation between undescended testis and renal agenesis.

Question 9.19: A 21-year-old male undergoes a scrotal ultrasound. The left testis is not visualized within the left hemiscrotum. The left groin is imaged and the key finding depicted in the image below. Which statement is correct?

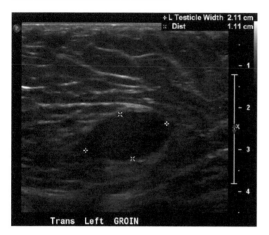

A The structure being measured is consistent with a groin lymph node.
B. There is a 30- to 50-fold increased risk of malignancy.
C. A biopsy is warranted.
D. If an underlying tumor develops, it would most likely be a Sertoli cell tumor.

Answer:
B. Correct. Undescended testis/cryptorchidism is associated with a 30- to 50-fold increased risk of malignancy, with seminoma and embryonal cell carcinoma accounting for the majority of cases.

A. Incorrect. Though a normal lymph node may be hypoechoic and oval in shape, the absence of the typical "echogenic hilum" allows the two entities to be distinguished.

C. Incorrect. If there are sufficient associated suspicious features, such as microlithiasis, an orchiectomy is indicated.

D. Incorrect. Seminoma and embryonal cell carcinoma account for the majority of malignancies in the setting of cryptorchidism.

Question 9.20: Images of the bilateral testes of a 34 year-old male are presented. The images demonstrate bilateral testicular masses. Which statement is correct with respect to bilateral testicular tumors?

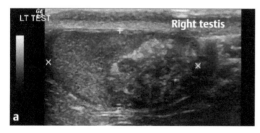

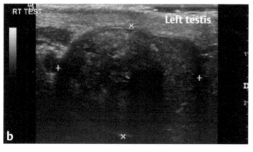

A. Synchronous tumors are more frequently encountered than metachronous tumors.
B. A testicular metastasis is more likely to arise from a contralateral testicular primary than from a distant primary.
C. Testicular lymphoma is bilateral in roughly 30% of cases.
D. None of the above.

Answer:
C. Correct. Testicular lymphoma is bilateral in up to 30% of cases.

A. Incorrect. Synchronous testicular tumors are much less common than metachronous tumors, with synchronous tumors accounting for only 10% of bilateral testicular tumors.

B. Incorrect. The testes do no share vascular and lymphatic connections, so a tumor in one testis is unlikely to spread to the other. Instead testicular metastases, though rare, likely arise from other primary sources such as the prostate.

D. Incorrect.

Question 9.21: Images of the bilateral testes of a 34 year-old male are presented. The images demonstrate bilateral testicular masses. Imaging of the upper abdomen of the patient revealed bilateral adrenal masses. What is the most appropriate management of this condition?

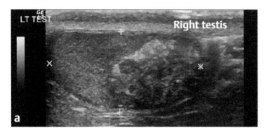

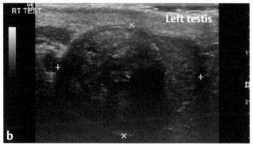

A. Percutaneous biopsy of the adrenal lesions.

B. Colonoscopy.

C. Chemotherapy and scrotal radiotherapy.

D. High-dose glucocorticoid therapy.

Answer:

D. Correct. The patient's testicular masses are adrenal rest tumors. Testicular adrenal rests are clusters of cells that become trapped within the developing gonad. These adrenal rests can be found in roughly 10% of newborns and about 2% of adults. They are typically asymptomatic, unless exposed to elevated levels of adrenocorticotropic hormone, in which case they enlarge to form masses. This patient has a history of congenital adrenal hyperplasia which led to stimulation of the adrenal rest. This condition may be treated with steroids.

A, B, C—Incorrect. These are not indicated.

Further Readings

Adham WK, Raval BK, Uzquiano MC, Lemos LB. Best cases from the AFIP: bilateral testicular tumors: seminoma and mixed germ cell tumor. Radiographics 2005;25(3):835–839

Coursey Moreno C, Small WC, Camacho JC, et al. Testicular tumors: what radiologists need to know—differential diagnosis, staging, and management. Radiographics 2015;35(2):400–415

Dogra VS, Gottlieb RH, Oka M, Rubens DJ. Sonography of the scrotum. Radiology 2003;227(1):18–36

Dogra VS, Gottlieb RH, Rubens DJ, Liao L. Benign intratesticular cystic lesions: US features. Radiographics 2001;21(Spec No):S273–S281

Frates MC, Benson CB, DiSalvo DN, Brown DL, Laing FC, Doubilet PM. Solid extratesticular masses evaluated with sonography: pathologic correlation. Radiology 1997;204(1):43–46

Garriga V, Serrano A, Marin A, Medrano S, Roson N, Pruna X. US of the tunica vaginalis testis: anatomic relationships and pathologic conditions. Radiographics 2009;29(7):2017–2032

Ishigami K, Abu-Yousef MM, El-Zein Y. Tubular ectasia of the epididymis: a sign of postvasectomy status. J Clin Ultrasound 2005;33(9):447–451

Jarraya M, Hayashi D, de Villiers RV, et al. Multimodality imaging of foreign bodies of the musculoskeletal system. AJR Am J Roentgenol 2014;203(1):W92-102

Loya AG, Said JW, Grant EG. Epidermoid cyst of the testis: radiologic-pathologic correlation. Radiographics 2004;24(Suppl 1):S243–S246

Woodward PJ, Schwab CM, Sesterhenn IA. From the archives of the AFIP: extratesticular scrotal masses: radiologic-pathologic correlation. Radiographics 2003;23(1):215–240

Chapter 10

Miscellaneous

Scott Stevens, Halemane Ganesh, and Adrian Dawkins

10 Questions and Answers

Question 10.1: This sonographic image below demonstrates a color Doppler overlay in the region of the main portal vein. What accounts for the incomplete color fill-in?

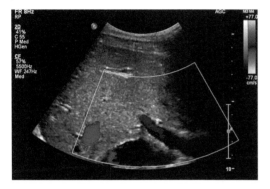

A. Nonocclusive thrombus.
B. Incorrect color priority setting.
C. Color box set too wide.
D. Color scale set too high.

Answer:
D. Correct. The color scale is set to +/-77 cm/second. When the color scale is set to this high value, there is also an unavoidable increase in the wall filter. This results in obscuration of low-velocity flow, hence the incomplete portal venous color fill-in.

A. Incorrect. The incomplete color fill-in is artifactual.

B. Incorrect. The color priority setting affects which shades of gray can be replaced by color, since the display has to choose between the grayscale and color. The color priority bar is seen as the progressively darkening band adjacent to the color bar. In this example, the color priority is set high (green line at top of band), therefore optimized for the detection of flow.

C. Incorrect. The color box should be positioned tightly around the structure being interrogated. In this example, there is perhaps opportunity to decrease the width; however, this measure would not improve the color fill-in.

Question 10.2: With reference to the image below, which statement is correct?

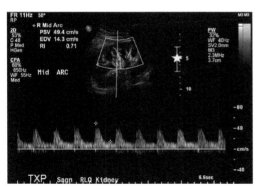

A. The angle correction is poorly aligned resulting in an inaccurate resistive index measurement.
B. The lack of any "blue" areas within the renal parenchyma suggests occlusion of the renal vein.

C. The resistive index is being measured incorrectly.
D. The beam is focused incorrectly.

Answer:
C. Correct. The resistive index is obtained by dividing the difference of the peak systolic velocity (PSV) and end diastolic velocity (EDV) by the PSV, that is, (PSV − EDV)/PSV. In this example, the second caliper is not positioned at the EDV, since the EDV occurs just before the sharp systolic upstroke. In the case presented, the error is perhaps not significant since the second half of the cycle is fairly flat. However, this is not always the case and significantly erroneous measurements could be obtained.

A. Incorrect. The resistive index measurement is not dependent on angle correction, since both the PSV and EDV will be affected by the same factor, cancelling out during calculation.

B. Incorrect. The color bar displays graded shades of pink, a frequent color assignment for power Doppler. Power Doppler typically yields no directional information but is very useful at demonstrating areas of slow flow. Consequently, when using this display setting, there will be no "blue" areas to indicate flow in the opposite direction.

D. Incorrect. The ultrasound beam is focused appropriately at the level of the renal parenchyma as illustrated by the focus position bar (*yellow star*).

Question 10.3: Regarding this image, which statement is correct?

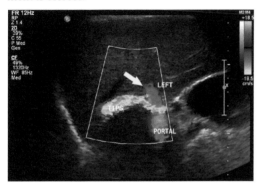

A. The findings are within normal limits.
B. Aliasing within the transjugular intrahepatic portosystemic shunt (TIPSS) is suggestive of malfunction.
C. The direction of flow within the left branch of the portal vein (*yellow arrow*) is suggestive of malfunction.
D. None of the above.

Answer:
A. Correct. The color scale (+/- 18.5 cm/second) has been optimized to demonstrate flow within the portal vein. However, as a result of this relatively low scale, there is commensurate aliasing within the TIPSS because of the normal higher velocities within the TIPSS (90–190 cm/second). Reversal of flow with the left branch of the portal vein is a sign of a proper functioning TIPSS.

B. Incorrect. Aliasing occurs because of the normal higher velocities within the TIPSS.

C. Incorrect. Reversal of flow within the left branch of the portal vein is a sign of a proper functioning TIPSS.

D. Incorrect.

Question 10.4: This 67-year-old patient presents with abdominal pain and undergoes an abdominal ultrasound. The patient's symptoms are likely worsened by which factor?

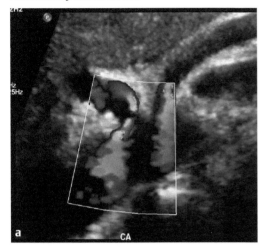

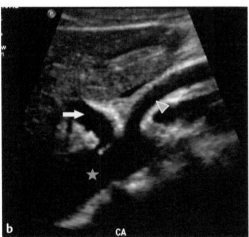

Answer:

B. Correct. The image demonstrates the celiac axis (*yellow arrow*) and superior mesenteric artery (*green arrow*) in the longitudinal plane, as they originate from the aorta (*star*). At grayscale, the celiac axis origin is seen to be severely narrowed. The color Doppler overlay reveals aliasing in this region. These findings are consistent with median arcuate ligament syndrome (MALS). This condition is exacerbated by in expiration.

A. Incorrect. The symptoms experienced in MALS are worsening by eating.

C. Incorrect. MALS is exacerbated by lying supine but somewhat alleviated by an erect posture.

D. Incorrect.

A. Fasting.
B. Expiration.
C. Erect posture.
D. None of the above.

Question 10.5: A 58-year-old male patient presents with elevated liver function tests. He was the recipient of a transplanted liver. What is suggested by this duplex evaluation at the porta hepatis.

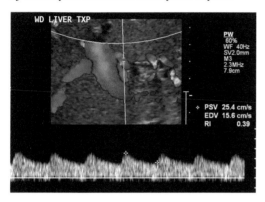

A. Hepatic artery stenosis.
B. Hepatic arterial occlusion.
C. Aneurysmal portal vein.
D. Reversed portal venous flow.

Answer:
A. Correct. The image reveals spectral Doppler evaluation of the hepatic artery. The obtained waveform reveals a prolonged acceleration time and decreased overall peak velocity resulting in the classic "parvus tardus" waveform. This is usually the result of proximal stenosis.

B. Incorrect. The hepatic artery is seen to be patent.

C. Incorrect. The portal vein is normal in caliber.

D. Incorrect. The directionality of the portal vein cannot be definitely inferred since the directionality color bar has been cropped (though the flow is known to be antegrade by the author). However, reversed portal venous flow in the setting of a liver transplant is very uncommon, often with a poor outcome.

Question 10.6: Which of the following is a complication that is associated with hepatic artery stenosis in a transplanted liver?
A. Portal hypertension.
B. Biliary necrosis.
C. Thromboembolic disease.
D. Splenic vein occlusion.

Answer:
B. Correct. In the setting of a liver transplant, the integrity of the biliary tree is dependent on the hepatic arterial circulation. If hepatic arterial stenosis is sufficiently severe, it may lead to biliary necrosis.

A. Incorrect. Portal hypertension is not directly associated with hepatic artery stenosis.

C. Incorrect. Thromboembolic disease is not directly associated with hepatic artery stenosis.

D. Incorrect. Splenic vein occlusion is not directly associated with hepatic artery stenosis.

Question 10.7: A 54-year-old male presents with repeated episodes of hematemesis and hematochezia. An ultrasound of the upper abdomen is performed, an image from which is presented below. How should the patient be definitively managed?

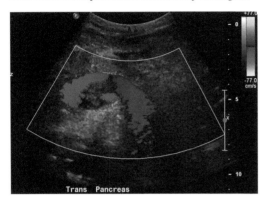

A. Splenectomy.
B. Thrombectomy.
C. Thrombolysis.
D. Placement of TIPSS.

Answer:

A. Correct. The image demonstrates incomplete color fill-in of the splenic vein consistent with splenic vein thrombosis (SVT). SVT is occasionally complicated by upper gastrointestinal bleeding secondary to esophageal varices. This is usually treated definitively with splenectomy, effectively removing the problematic collateral pathway.

B. Incorrect. Thrombectomy is at best a temporizing measure.

C. Incorrect. Thrombolysis is at best a temporizing measure.

D. Incorrect. A TIPSS may be undertaken in patients with intractable upper gastrointestinal bleeding. However, extensive SVT, possibly extending to the portal vein often renders a TIPSS ineffective.

Question 10.8: What finding is depicted?

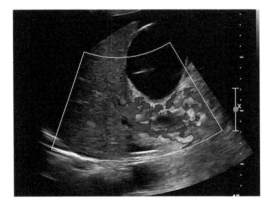

A. Cavernous transformation of the portal vein.
B. Aneurysmal portal vein.
C. Arteriovenous shunt.
D. Budd–Chiari syndrome.

Answer:

A. Correct. The images demonstrate occlusion of the main portal vein with multiple surrounding small collateral vessels. These finding represent cavernous transformation of the portal vein usually the result of longstanding portal hypertension.

B. Incorrect. An aneurysmal portal vein is not imaged.

C. Incorrect. Arterioportal shunts are usually observed as intrahepatic nodular enhancing foci on cross-sectional imaging.

D. Incorrect. Budd–Chiari syndrome usually manifests as marked enlargement of the caudate lobe and nonvisualization of the hepatic veins.

Question 10.9: The complex fluid collection superior to this transplanted kidney (*arrow*) was proven to be a hematoma. What other clinically pertinent finding is present?

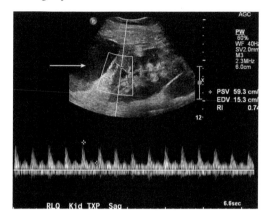

A. Borderline elevated resistive index.

B. Absence of renal venous flow.

C. Concerning physiologic response.

D. Increased PSV of parenchymal vessels.

Answer:

C. Correct. The image demonstrates marked tachycardia, calculated by counting the peaks within the time scale outlined at the bottom of the image. The time scale indicates roughly 6 seconds, within which there are approximately 14 peaks. Consequently, the heart rate is about 140 beats/minute. Observing the pattern of the spectral tracing can often reveal clinically useful information such as arrhythmias.

A. Incorrect. The resistive index (0.74) is within normal limits.

B. Incorrect. Absent renal venous flow would manifest as reversed arterial diastolic flow.

D. Incorrect. PSV should be interpreted with caution since reliable angle correction is challenging when evaluating very small vessels.

Question 10.10: A 46-year-old male is to be discharged 2 days post TIPSS placement for refractory ascites. The clinical service requests an ultrasound study to confirm TIPSS patency prior to discharge. A representative image from this study is demonstrated below. Based on the appearances, which management strategy is correct.

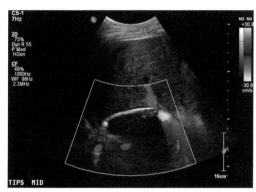

A. Repeat angiography to confirm patency, even if there are no clinical signs of TIPSS occlusion.

B. Initiate thrombolytic therapy.

C. Repeat ultrasound in 1 week.

D. None of the above.

Answer:

C. Correct. Soon after the deployment of some TIPSS devices, in particular covered stents, air may become trapped within the expanding wall, rendering evaluation of patency invalid. One key clue to artifactual occlusion is the inability to visualize the far wall of the device, as in this case. It typically takes 1 week for the gas to dissipate so, unless there is a clinical concern regarding patency, some shunts are best evaluated at least 1 week post placement.

A. Incorrect. This measure would be unnecessary.

B. Incorrect. This measure would be unnecessary and inappropriate.

D. Incorrect.

Question 10.11: Regarding carotid ultrasound, the sonographic maneuver annotated TT below is most often used to identify which vessel?

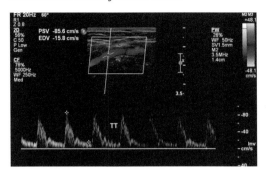

A. Internal carotid artery (ICA).
B. External carotid artery (ECA).
C. Common carotid artery (CCA).
D. Vertebral artery (VA).

Answer:

B. Correct. TT refers to "temporal tap" as is obtained by tapping over the superficial temporal artery while interrogating the ECA. This transmitted thrill can be seen as a saw-tooth appearance. This helps to confirm that the ECA is being evaluated as opposed to the closely related ICA since the superficial temporal artery is a branch of the ECA.

A, C, D—Incorrect. The temporal tap maneuver is used to identify the ECA.

Question 10.12: Regarding carotid ultrasound, which of the imaging parameters below is most often the best for grading the severity of cervical carotid stenoses?

A. PSV in the ICA.
B. EDV in the ICA.
C. PSV in the CCA.
D. ICA/CCA PSV ratio.

Answer:

A. Correct. Primary parameters for estimating the degree of stenosis include the PSV and visible plaque.

B, C—Incorrect. These measures are not useful for estimating stenosis.

D. Incorrect. The ICA/CCA PSV ratio is a secondary parameter but may be of value when overall carotid velocities are elevated, say in hypertension.

Question 10.13: A 71-year-old diabetic male presents with right foot pain. An ultrasound is performed as shown. What finding is highly suggestive of distal occlusion?

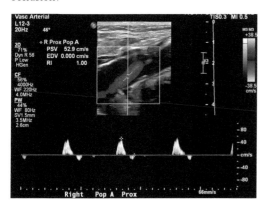

A. Incomplete color fill-in.

B. Spectral broadening.

C. Aliasing.

D. Loss of the majority of diastolic flow.

Answer:

D. Correct. A normal popliteal artery would demonstrate vascular flow throughout the cardiac cycle, often creating a triphasic waveform. In this case, the peak velocity is marginally diminished and there is loss of the majority of diastolic flow. This has been described as the preocclusive "thump" or "staccato" waveform indicating a distal occlusion.

A. Incorrect. Incomplete color fill-in suggests thrombus at the site of interrogation.

B. Incorrect. Spectral broadening (filling in of the spectral curve) is also suggestive of stenosis at the site of interrogation.

C. Incorrect. Aliasing may be encountered within stenotic segments of vessels due to increased velocity. However, aliasing does not necessarily indicate a distal occlusion.

Question 10.14: This image is obtained from a patient with Gaucher's disease. Which statement is correct?

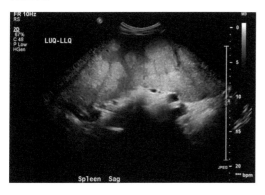

A. Splenomegaly is an uncommon manifestation.

B. When hyperechoic lesions are present within the spleen, splenectomy is recommended.

C. Thrombocytopenia is a complication of this condition.

D. Splenic lesions in the setting of Gaucher's disease are highly suggestive of lymphoma.

Answer:

C. Correct. Gaucher's disease is a lysosomal storage disorder resulting in the accumulation of glucocerebroside within lysosomes of mononuclear phagocytes. This typically affects the bone marrow, liver, and spleen. The spleen is typically enlarged and may demonstrate several focal lesions which may be hypo- or hyperechoic on ultrasound. "Gaucheromas" may also be present within the liver. These lesions demonstrate no known malignant potential and, though of indeterminate etiology, may result from a combination of infarction, extramedullary hematopoiesis, and fibrosis. Thrombocytopenia is known complication of Gaucher's disease.

A. Incorrect. Splenomegaly is typically present.

B. Incorrect. This would be an unnecessary measure.

D. Incorrect. These lesions are unlikely to represent lymphoma.

Question 10.15: Sonographic images of the spleen were obtained in an 8-year-old patient with bruising. What is the likely diagnosis?

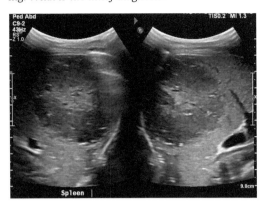

A.   Hemangioma.
B.   Angiosarcoma.
C.   Hamartoma.
D.   Lymphangioma.

Answer:

A. Correct. The images represent a path-proven large splenic hemangioma. Large hemangiomas have a propensity to bleed. Also, there may be associated consumptive coagulopathy predisposing the patient to bleeds, for example, Kasabach–Merritt syndrome.

B. Incorrect. Splenic angiosarcomas are exceedingly rare and tend to occur in the middle-aged individuals. Ultrasound appearances are nonspecific.

C. Incorrect. Splenic hamartomas are uncommon lesions that tend to be hyperechoic with respect to the background splenic parenchyma. Bruising is not typically associated with splenic hamartomas.

D. Incorrect. Splenic lymphangiomas tend to occur in children but are typically cystic in morphology.

Question 10.16: The splenic lesion imaged below is consistent with which of the following?

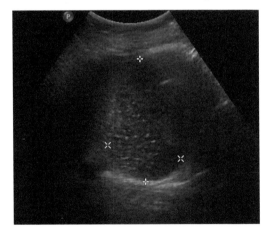

A.   An infarct.
B.   An abscess.
C.   A granuloma.
D.   A metastatic deposit.

Answer 10.16:

A. Correct. The image demonstrates a wedge-shaped somewhat reticulated area of hypoechogenicity within the splenic parenchyma. This finding is typical of a splenic infarct.

B. Incorrect. Infarcts may progress to abscess formation. However, an abscess typically manifests as a complex fluid collection with surrounding hyperemia.

C. Incorrect. A granuloma typically presents as a punctate echogenic focus consistent with calcification. They are often multiple.

D. Incorrect. Splenic metastases are relatively uncommon but would typically present as a hypoechoic rounded lesion.

Question 10.17: What is the likely cause for this appearance in this 17-year-old African American patient with abdominal pain and anemia?

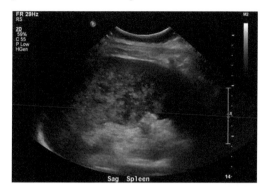

A. Splenic sequestration.
B. Echinococcal disease.
C. Splenic abscess.
D. Gamna–Gandy bodies.

Answer 10.17:

A. Correct. This patient has a history of sickle cell anemia. The spleen is larger than expected for age, since 94% of HbSS patients are "asplenic" by the age of 5 years. The heterogenous appearance of the splenic parenchyma is typical of splenic sequestration, the result of trapping of red blood cells within the spleen. Early recognition of the finding is vital to limit adverse outcomes.

B. Incorrect. Echinococcal disease of the spleen usually results in the formation of "hydatid cysts" which may vary from solitary cysts to a dominant cystic lesion with contained daughter cysts.

C. Incorrect. An abscess would manifest as a complex fluid collection with surrounding hyperemia. Gas may also be contained.

D. Incorrect. Gamna–Gandy bodies represent foci of microhemorrhage within the spleen and usually signify portal hypertension. These lesions are usually diagnosed on in-and-out of phase T1-weighted magnetic resonance images. Sonographically these lesions are frequently occult. Occasionally, Gamna–Gandy bodies are seen as punctate echogenic foci throughout the spleen, with or without acoustic shadowing.

Question 10.18: A patient presents with a history of recurrent abdominal pain. An ultrasound is undertaken. The width of which structure is being measured?

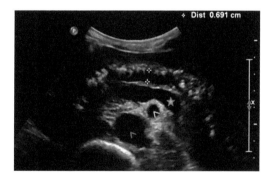

A. Pancreatic duct.
B. Left renal vein.
C. Splenic vein.
D. Common bile duct.

Answer:

A. Correct. The image demonstrates a tubular structure with numerous associated echogenic foci. This tubular structure is anterior to the splenic vein (*star*). The findings are consistent with a dilated pancreatic duct.

B. Incorrect. The left renal vein runs between the superior mesenteric artery (*yellow arrow*) and the aorta (*blue arrow*). It is not imaged.

C. Incorrect. The splenic vein is indicated by the *star*.

D. Incorrect. The distal portion of the common bile duct may be visualized as it traverses the pancreatic head. It is not imaged.

Question 10.19: What is the likely diagnosis of the patient in (Question 10.18)?

A. Splenorenal shunt.

B. Chronic pancreatitis.

C. Nonocclusive thrombosis of the splenic vein.

D. Choledocholithiasis.

Answer:

B. Correct. The combination of a dilated pancreatic duct and numerous parenchymal and ductal punctate calcifications are consistent with changes of chronic pancreatitis.

A. Incorrect. A splenorenal shunt is frequently encountered in portal hypertension, allowing blood to return to the right heart via the left renal vein and inferior vena cava, bypassing the portal circulation. Such a shunt is not imaged.

C. Incorrect. The splenic vein is patent.

D. Incorrect. The common bile duct is not imaged.

Question 10.20: A 36-year-old female presents with abdominal pain. The structure labeled "a" is?

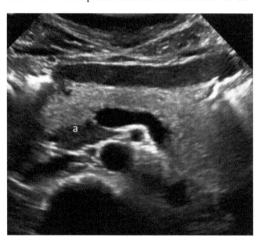

A. Consistent with focal acute pancreatitis.

B. Consistent with a pancreatic neoplasm.

C. A peripancreatic lymph node.

D. A normal variant.

Answer:

D. Correct. The image demonstrates a well-defined area of relative hypoechogenicity involving the ventral pancreas. This is a normal variant due to relatively less fat content within the ventral pancreas as compared to the remaining pancreatic parenchyma.

A. Incorrect. The pancreas is often sonographically normal in the seating of generalized or focal pancreatitis.

B. Incorrect. A pancreatic neoplasm may be seen as a distinct mass within the pancreas, often with pancreatic ductal dilation.

C. Incorrect. A lymph node would be seen as a separate oval-shaped structure.

Question 10.21: A 36-year-old female presents with a history of abdominal pain. A longitudinal sonographic view of the upper abdomen is presented below. What is the likely underlying cause for finding indicated by the *arrow*?

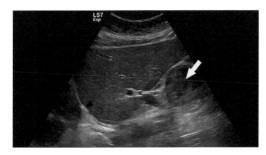

A. Serous cystadenoma.

B. Solid pseudopapillary epithelial neoplasm (SPEN).

C. Acute necrotic collection.

D. Walled-off necrosis.

Answer:

B. Correct. The *arrow* indicates a mixed solid and cystic lesion in the expected location of the pancreatic head. Of the choices provided, a SPEN is the most likely diagnosis, typically occurring in young female adults (third decade of life). This benign lesion is frequently noted to be solid with cystic areas.

A. Incorrect. A serous cystadenoma also demonstrates a female predilection, though in an older demographic. Also, these lesions are typically more cystic in morphology than demonstrated in this case.

C. Incorrect. An acute necrotic collection occurs as a complication of acute pancreatitis. This lesion would be predominantly cystic, unlike this case.

D. Incorrect. Walled-off necrosis occurs as a complication of acute pancreatitis. As above, this lesion would be predominantly cystic, unlike this case.

Further Readings

Atri M, Nazarnia S, Mehio A, Reinhold C, Bret PM. Hypoechogenic embryologic ventral aspect of the head and uncinate process of the pancreas: in vitro correlation of US with histopathologic findings. Radiology 1994;190(2):441–444

Bhatt S, Simon R, Dogra VS. Gamna-Gandy bodies: sonographic features with histopathologic correlation. J Ultrasound Med 2006;25(12):1625–1629

Darcy M. Evaluation and management of transjugular intrahepatic portosystemic shunts. AJR Am J Roentgenol 2012;199(4):730–736

Grant EG, Benson CB, Moneta GL, et al. Carotid artery stenosis: gray-scale and Doppler US diagnosis—Society of Radiologists in Ultrasound Consensus Conference. Radiology 2003;229(2):340–346

Hoeger PH, Helmke K, Winkler K. Chronic consumption coagulopathy due to an occult splenic haemangioma: Kasabach-Merritt syndrome. Eur J Pediatr 1995;154(5): 365–368

Kruskal JB, Newman PA, Sammons LG, Kane RA. Optimizing Doppler and color flow US: application to hepatic sonography. Radiographics 2004;24(3):657–675

Lonergan GJ, Cline DB, Abbondanzo SL. Sickle cell anemia. Radiographics 2001;21(4):971–994

Poll LW, Vom Dahl S. Image of the month. Hepatic Gaucheroma mimicking focal nodular hyperplasia. Hepatology 2009;50(3):985–986

Stein P, Malhotra A, Haims A, Pastores GM, Mistry PK. Focal splenic lesions in type I Gaucher disease are associated with poor platelet and splenic response to macrophage-targeted enzyme replacement therapy. J Inherit Metab Dis 2010;33(6):769–774

Sunkara S, Williams TR, Myers DT, Kryvenko ON. Solid pseudopapillary tumours of the pancreas: spectrum of imaging findings with histopathological correlation. Br J Radiol 2012;85(1019):e1140–e1144

Tembey RA, Bajaj AS, Wagle PK, Ansari AS. Real-time ultrasound: Key factor in identifying celiac artery compression syndrome. Indian J Radiol Imaging 2015;25(2):202–205

Chapter 11

Physics

Gary Ge and Adrian Dawkins

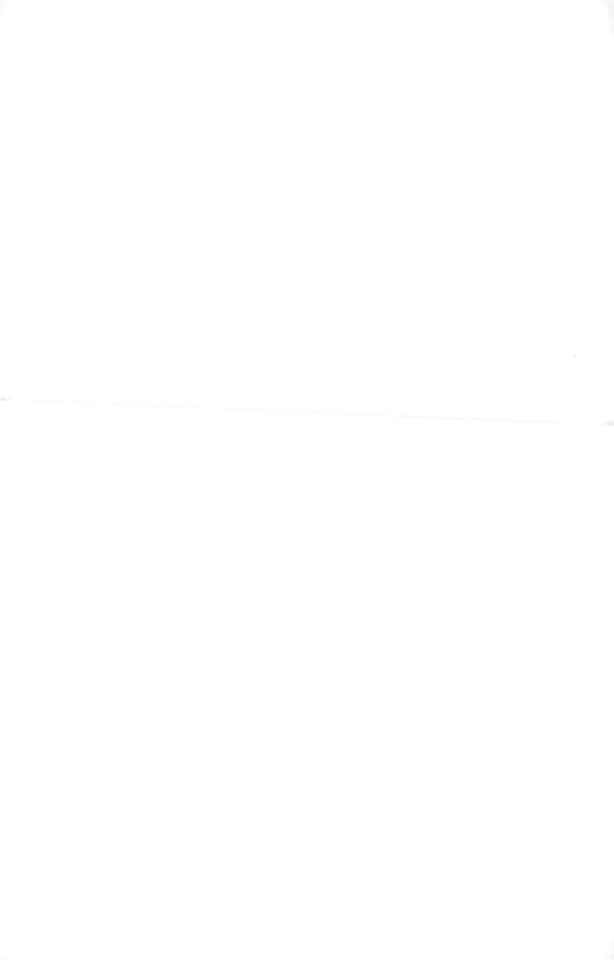

11 Questions and Answers

Question 11.1: If the amplitude of the ultrasound beam is attenuated by a factor of 2 (halved), the intensity will be changed by what factor?

A. ¼.

B. ½.

C. 2.

D. 4.

Answer:

A. Correct. The intensity of an ultrasound beam is proportional to the square of the amplitude.

B, C, D—Incorrect. Intensity is proportional to the square of the amplitude.

Question 11.2: If the operating frequency is changed from 5 to 2.5 MHz, the wavelength will?

A. Decrease by a factor of 2.

B. Increase by a factor of 2.

C. Decrease by a factor of 4.

D. Increase by a factor of 4.

Answer:

B. Correct. The wavelength of a sound wave is inversely related to frequency in any uniform medium as shown by the equation:

$$\text{velocity} = \text{frequency} \times \text{wavelength}.$$

A, C, D—Incorrect. Wavelength is inversely related to frequency.

Question 11.3: The "matching layer" within an ultrasound transducer should ideally have a thickness of?

A. One-fourth the wavelength of the probe's sound wave.

B. Half the wavelength of the probe's sound wave.

C. Three-fourth the wavelength of the probe's sound wave.

D. One wavelength of the probe's sound wave.

Answer:

A. Correct. The matching layer is used to minimize the large acoustic impedance (AI) mismatch between the transducer's crystal and the patient's tissue. Recall that a large AI mismatch between two materials results in very little transmission of sound across the interface of the materials, that is, the sound is largely reflected. Therefore, the matching layer facilitates transmission of sound which is necessary for imaging. The ideal thickness of the matching layer is one-fourth the wavelength, simply because this results in a net cancelation of any interfering sound from the matching layer itself.

B, C, D—Incorrect. The ideal thickness of the matching layer is one-fourth the wavelength.

Question 11.4: Which statement is true?

A. The thickness of a transducer crystal is half the wavelength of the sound it creates.

B. The thickness of a transducer crystal is equal to the wavelength of the sound it creates.

C. The thickness of a transducer crystal is twice the wavelength of the sound it produces.

D. None of the above.

Answer:

A. Correct. The thicker the crystal, the larger the wavelength and hence the lower the frequency. Recall, $f \propto 1/\lambda$.

B, C, D—Incorrect. The thickness of a transducer crystal is half the wavelength of the sound it creates.

Question 11.5: Sound travels faster in muscle than fat. How does a 10-MHz beam change as it travels from fat to muscle?
A. The amplitude increases.
B. Frequency increases.
C. Wavelength increases.
D. None of the above.

Answer:
C. Correct. According to the equation for the speed of sound ($v = f \times \lambda$), an increase in speed causes a linear increase in wavelength since the frequency stays the same.

A. Incorrect. The amplitude is not necessarily altered.

B. Incorrect. The frequency stays the same.

D. Incorrect. The wavelength increases.

Question 11.6: If the diameter of an ultrasound transducer is doubled, the focal spot distance will?
A. Increase by a factor of 8.
B. Increase by a factor of 4.
C. Decrease by a factor of 8.
D. Decrease by a factor of 4.

Answer:
B. Correct. The distance from the transducer to the focal spot is defined by the equation:

$$\text{Near field length} = \frac{d^2}{4\lambda}$$

where d is the diameter and λ is the wavelength. Doubling the diameter results in a 4-fold increase since $(2d)^2 = 4d^2$.

A, C, D—Incorrect. Near field length is related to the square of the diameter of the transducer.

Question 11.7: Which tissue interface results in the largest amount of sound reflection?
A. Soft tissue/liver.
B. Air/fat.
C. Bone/muscle.
D. Muscle/soft tissue.

Answer:
B. Correct. The acoustic impedance (AI) of air is so small that boundaries with air and any tissue result in nearly 100% reflection of the sound beam. This is why ultrasound gel is required for scanning, as it facilitates some transmission.

A, C, D—Incorrect. Boundaries with air and any tissue result in nearly 100% reflection of the sound beam.

Question 11.8: What change in decibel (dB) is represented by a 50% loss in beam intensity?
A. 0.5 dB.
B. 3 dB.
C. 5 dB.
D. 10 dB.

Answer:
B. Correct. The equation for dB is as follows: dB = $10 \log (I/I_0)$ where I_0 is the original intensity and I is the new intensity. If there is a 50% loss in intensity then the change in dB = 10 (log 50/100) = 10 (log 0.5) = 10 (− 0.3) = −3. Note that doubling the intensity results in the same dB change, that is, 10 (log 2) = 10 (0.3) = 3. Clearly a negative change indicates a decrease while a positive change indicates an increase.

A, C, D—Incorrect. A halving or doubling of the intensity is reflected by a 3 dB change.

Question 11.9: What is the fundamental frequency of the harmonic mode for an ultrasound exam with a 3-MHz transducer?

A.   3 MHz.

B.   6 MHz.

C.   9 MHz.

D.   12 MHz.

Answer:

A. Correct. The fundamental frequency for harmonic imaging refers to the center frequency of the ultrasound transducer which is 3-MHz in this case.

B, C, D—Incorrect. The fundamental frequency refers to the center frequency.

Question 11.10: What is the typical contrast bubble size for ultrasound imaging?

A.   1 to 5 μm.

B.   15 to 25 μm.

C.   35 to 45 μm.

D.   55 to 65 μm.

Answer:

A. Correct. Contrast bubbles are normally between 1 and 5 μm, about the size of a red blood corpuscle.

B, C, D—Incorrect. Contrast bubbles are normally between 1 and 5 μm.

Question 11.11: Which of the following is not true of microbubble technology?

A.   Once injected, microbubbles remain confined to the vascular compartment until degradation.

B.   Microbubbles typically degrade after 4 to 6 minutes.

C.   The inert gas, within the core of the microbubbles, is excreted via the urinary tract, though not discernible to the patient.

D.   High mechanical index (MI) settings will destroy microbubbles.

Answer:

C. Correct. Microbubbles are injected intravenously and remain within the intravascular compartment until degradation, typically 4 to 6 minutes after injection. The gas within the core of the bubbles is excreted via the lungs. A low MI setting is required to preserve the integrity of the bubbles since high MI settings lead to accelerated degradation.

A, B, D—Incorrect. These statements are true.

Question 11.12: A 6-MHz ultrasound beam is used to produce an image from a structure at a depth of 15 cm within soft tissue. The image is suboptimal and a 4-MHz probe was used to improve the imaging. How much less attenuation is experienced with the 4-MHz probe?

A.   2 dB.

B.   15 dB.

C.   30 dB.

D.   60 dB.

Answer:

C. Correct. Using the rule of thumb that an ultrasound beam is attenuated 0.5 dB/MHz/cm, a 6-MHz beam will be attenuated by 90 dB over the 30 cm (to and fro) journey. A 4-MHz beam will be attenuated by 60 dB. The difference is, therefore, 30 dB. From a practical standpoint, a decrease of 3 dB equates to a weakening of the original beam by 50%. Therefore, the difference of 30 dB equates to a 50% weakening ten times (recall 30 = 3 × 10).

A, B, D—Incorrect. An ultrasound beam is attenuated 0.5 dB/MHz/cm.

Question 11.13: While traveling through which of the following materials does ultrasound experience the most attenuation?

A. Soft tissue.

B. Lung.

C. Bone.

D. Muscle.

Answer:

B. Correct. Lungs have the highest attenuation coefficient for tissue of around 40 dB/cm for a 1-MHz beam, followed by bone which is approximately 20 dB/cm. Other tissues are generally close to 1 dB/cm.

A. Incorrect. This is generally closer to 1 dB/cm.

C. Incorrect. Lung typically has the highest attenuation coefficient of around 40 dB/cm for a 1-MHz beam, followed by bone which is approximately 20 dB/cm.

D. Incorrect. This is generally closer to 1 dB/cm.

Question 11.14: Which of the time gain compensation (TGC) curves is associated with highest transducer frequency?

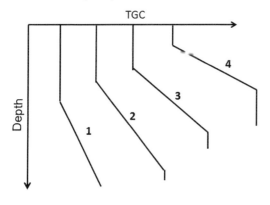

A. 1.

B. 2.

C. 3.

D. 4.

Answer:

D. Correct. The highest transducer frequency experiences the largest attenuation in a propagating medium, thus requiring the value of the TGC to be larger in order to accurately compensate the loss of signal intensity. Curve 4 demonstrates this correctly as it has the steepest TGC increase and the increase begins at the shallowest depth.

A, B, C—Incorrect. These are not associated with the highest transducer frequency.

Question 11.15: Reverberation artifact may be eliminated by changing which parameter?

A. Transducer frequency.

B. Transducer orientation.

C. Time gain compensation.

D. Pulse repetition period.

Answer:

B. Correct. Reverberation artifact is caused by two closely spaced interfaces that reflect sound back and forth during the acquisition of signal. Since specific angles create the artifact, it can often be eliminated by changing the transducer orientation.

A, C, D—Incorrect. These measures would not be effective in removing the artifact.

Question 11.16: The scanning scenario (**a**) results in image (**b**). What accounts for the difference?

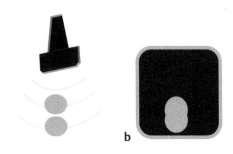

a   b

A. Suboptimal lateral resolution.
B. Suboptimal axial resolution.
C. Suboptimal receiver gain.
D. None of the above.

Answer:
B. Correct. The axial resolution is a measure of the system's ability to separate two closely positioned structures along the same vertical scan line. The axial resolution improves with increasing transducer frequency.

A. Incorrect. The lateral resolution is a measure of the system's ability to separate two closely positioned structures lying side by side. The lateral resolution improves with decreasing beam width.

C. Incorrect. Increasing the receiver gain will brighten the displayed image but not improve the signal-to-noise ratio or resolution.

D. Incorrect. The axial resolution improves with increasing transducer frequency.

Question 11.17: An ultrasound image is showing up too dark on the monitor. What adjustment to the scanning parameters should be made first to fix the issue?
A. Increase output power.
B. Increase receiver gain.
C. Decrease output power.
D. Decrease receiver gain.

Answer:
B. Correct. Increasing receiver gain and output power will both increase the brightness of the image, however adjusting the receiver gain is preferable because increasing output power will deposit more energy within the patient.

A. Incorrect. Increasing the output power would deposit more energy within the patient and is therefore not the best choice.

C, D—Incorrect. These measures would worsen the appearance.

Question 11.18: While performing an ultrasound of the right upper quadrant, the technologist notices a rounded hyperechoic focus above the diaphragm. What should he do next?

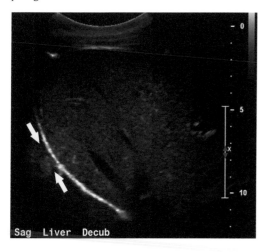

A. Change the angle of insonation.
B. Scan the other lung.
C. Turn up the overall gain.
D. Scan both kidneys.

Answer:
A. Correct. The finding above the diaphragm is a result of mirror artifact and characterized by a mirrored object about a strong reflector, in this case the lung–diaphragm interface. Changing the angle of insonation may help mitigate against this phenomenon.

B, C, D—Incorrect. These measures would not be effective in removing the artifact.

Question 11.19: A longitudinal view of the abdominal aorta is demonstrated below with a color Doppler overlay. What accounts for the two blue regions?

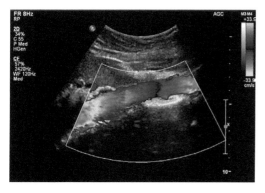

A. Hypertension.
B. Flow reversal.
C. Aortic stenosis.
D. None of the above.

Answer:
D. Correct. The blue region to the right of the screen, within the more distal aorta, produces a negative Doppler shift based on its orientation with the probe, as it arches away. Notice that the change from red to blue goes through "black" which indicates a true change in direction with respect to the angle of insonation. The blue region to the left of the screen occurs because this segment of the aorta is deeper and hence overwhelms the pulse repetition frequency (PRF), resulting in aliasing. Aliasing represents a misrepresentation of flow direction due to an inadequate sampling rate. Notice that the change from red to blue goes through "white" when aliasing occurs.

A. Incorrect. This does not account for the findings.

B. Incorrect. This does not completely account for the findings.

C. Incorrect. This does not account for the findings.

Question 11.20: Where is the beam narrowest?

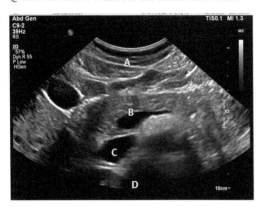

A. A.

B. B.

C. C.

D. D.

Answer:

B. Correct. Marker B is positioned at the depth of the focusing bar ("I"-shaped icon to the right of the image). This indicates the "waist" of the beam, where the focusing is optimized.

A, C, D—Incorrect. The beam is narrowest where focusing is optimized.

Question 11.21: How long did it take for position D to be interrogated by the sound beam? Refer to the image in (Question 11.20).

A. 130 μs.

B. 230 μs.

C. 360 μs.

D. 490 μs.

Answer:

A. Correct. Marker D is positioned at a depth of 10 cm. In imaging, sound typically takes 13 μs to make a 1 cm to and fro roundtrip. Therefore, at a depth of 10 cm, the round-trip would take roughly 130 μs.

B, C, D—Incorrect. The round-trip would take roughly 130 μs.

Question 11.22: Regarding pulse wave imaging, the duty factor is?

A. The percentage of time that the bean is "on."

B. The duration of a pulse.

C. The duration between two pulses.

D. The number of pulses per second.

Answer:

A. Correct. The duty factor describes the percentage of time that the transducer is emitting sound waves as opposed to receiving sound, during pulse wave imaging. It is frequently expressed as a percentage.

B. Incorrect. The duration of a pulse is the actual time the beam is on for each pulse (in μs).

C. Incorrect. The duration between pulses is the termed the "listening time."

D. Incorrect. This describes the PRF.

Question 11.23: Cavitation is more likely to occur in which of the following ultrasound examinations?

A. Two-dimensional imaging using harmonics.

B. Three-dimensional imaging.

C. Pulse wave Doppler.

D. Continuous-wave Doppler.

Answer:

D. Correct. Continuous-wave Doppler produces the highest beam intensity with a "duty factor" of 100%. The duty factor is the percentage of time that the beam is "on" meaning the rate of energy deposition can be much higher than any other imaging technique.

A, B, C—Incorrect. Continuous-wave Doppler produces the highest beam intensity and hence is more likely to cause cavitation.

Question 11.24: Which of the following ultrasound examinations would result in the greatest rise in temperature?

A. Scanning a prostate.

B. Scanning a kidney.

C. Scanning a fetus.

D. Scanning a bladder.

Answer:

C. Correct. Ultrasound examinations of anatomy containing tissue–bone interfaces have the largest thermal index (TI). Obstetric scanning is therefore most susceptible.

A, B, D—Incorrect. Ultrasound examinations of anatomy containing tissue-bone interfaces have the largest TI.

Question 11.25: While performing an abdominal ultrasound scan, the transducer accidentally falls to the floor. The transducer is retrieved, cleaned, and scanning is resumed. However, soon after, the technologist notices a slender crack within the casing. What action should be taken?

A. The technologist should stop scanning immediately and switch to a replacement transducer if available.

B. The technologist can safely complete the scan but should avoid placing gel directly within the crack.

C. The technologist should listen for any audible ringing, as this could indicate imminent overheating which could pose a risk to the patient.

D. The technologist should apply a probe cover and continue with the study.

Answer:

A. Correct. Patients undergoing diagnostic ultrasound examinations come into physical contact with electronic components of the machine including the cables and transducers. Under normal operating conditions, the transducer poses the greatest risk of exposing patients to electrical hazards. If the transducer casing is cracked, the sonographer should stop using it immediately since a cracked transducer casing may lead to electrical injury.

B, C, D—Incorrect. These actions would be inappropriate.

Question 11.26: A technologist is about to begin a pelvic scan utilizing a transvaginal probe. Prior to use, the transducer should be?

A. Sterilized using dry heat.

B. Sterilized using moist heat.

C. Disinfected using a chemical agent.

D. Disinfected using clean water.

Answer:

C. Correct. Transducers are typically disinfected between patients. This is typically achieved with a liquid disinfectant applied via wipes or immersion.

Endocavitary probes should undergo high-level disinfection between patients. Transducers are not sterilized.

A, B—Incorrect. Heating a transducer may damage the piezoelectric elements. Also, transducers are not typically sterilized between patients.

D. Water does not adequately disinfect.

Question 11.27: The Curie temperature or Curie point of piezoelectric materials is in the range of?
A. 100 to 200°C.
B. 200 to 300°C.
C. 300 to 400°C.
D. 400 to 500°C.

Answer:
C. Correct. The Curie point of the piezoelectric materials within ultrasound transducers is generally around 360°C. Beyond this temperature, the material becomes depolarized and loses its piezoelectric properties.

A, B, D—Incorrect. The Curie point is generally around 360 °C.

Question 11.28: Side lobe artifact occurs when?
A. Off axis energy encounters a strong reflector.
B. Off axis energy encounters a weak reflector.
C. Sound waves are repeatedly reflected between two highly reflective surfaces.
D. Sound waves are repeatedly reflected in a tetrahedron of air bubbles.

Answer:
A. Correct. In addition to the main axis beam, radial expansion of piezoelectric crystals creates low energy off axis beams, described as side lobes. If this off axis beam encounters a strong reflector, it may generate an echo that is received by the transducer and artifactually placed along the axis of the main beam. Side lobe artifact is usually encountered in anechoic structures such as the urinary bladder and gallbladder and most commonly seen with linear array transducers.

B. Incorrect. A strong reflector is required.

C. Incorrect. This describes reverberation artifact.

D. Incorrect. This describes ring-down artifact.

Question 11.29: How could the artifact in the image below be minimized?

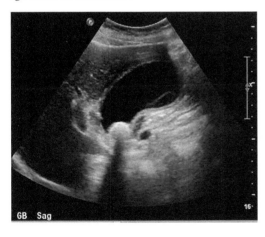

GB Sag

A. By increasing the frequency of the transducer.
B. By increasing the receiver gain.
C. By using spatial compounding.
D. By using harmonic imaging.

Answer:
C. Correct. The image shows posterior acoustic shadowing from a gallbladder calculus. The calculus attenuates sound to a greater degree than the surrounding structures, therefore the intensity of the beam distal to the calculus is weaker than the surrounding field. The attenuation worsens with increasing frequency. Shadowing decreases with spatial compounding and using multiple focal zones.

A. Incorrect. Shadowing worsens with increasing frequency.

B. Incorrect. This does not specifically affect the degree of shadowing.

D. Incorrect. Harmonic imaging results in better visualization of acoustic shadows.

Question 11.30: What accounts for the difference in the measured velocity within these two images obtained from the same patient during the same scan?

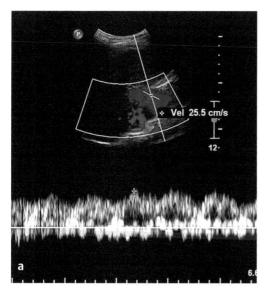

a

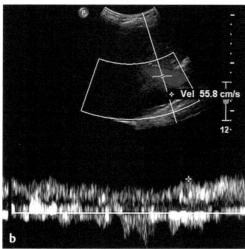

b

A. Angle of insonation.
B. Angle correction.
C. Beam focusing.
D. Color gain.

Answer:

B. Correct. The Doppler equation (below) reveals the inverse relationship between measured velocity (vel) and the cosine of the angle on insonation (cos θ). The machine must be "told" the angle at which the vessel is oriented while being interrogated. This is done by manually "correcting" the angle by aligning the angle indicator with the plane of the vessel. This is done fairly accurately in image **(a)** but overestimated in image **(b)**. Overestimating the angle results in an overestimation of the velocity since as θ increases from 0 to 90 degrees, cos θ decreases, making the denominator smaller and hence the velocity larger.

$$C \times f_{Dop} = vel\ f_0 \times 2 \times \cos \theta$$

A. Incorrect. The angle of insonation, that is, where the probe is positioned on the patient, is fairly constant across images (**a** and **b**).

C. Incorrect. This is fairly constant across images (**a** and **b**).

D. Incorrect. This is fairly constant across images (**a** and **b**).

Further Readings

Bushberg JT, Boone JM. The Essential Physics of Medical Imaging. Wolters Kluwer Health; 2011

Choudhry S, Gorman B, Charboneau JW, et al. Comparison of tissue harmonic imaging with conventional US in abdominal disease. Radiographics 2000;20(4):1127–1135

Feldman MK, Katyal S, Blackwood MSUS. US artifacts. Radiographics 2009;29(4):1179–1189

Hedrick WR, Hykes DL, Starchman DE. Ultrasound Physics and Instrumentation. Elsevier Mosby; 2005

Kremkau FW, Taylor KJ. Artifacts in ultrasound imaging. J Ultrasound Med 1986;5(4):227–237

Kremkau FW. Sonography Principles and Instruments. Elsevier Health Sciences; 2015

Pang EHT, Chan A, Ho SG, Harris AC. Contrast-enhanced ultrasound of the liver: optimizing technique and clinical applications. AJR Am J Roentgenol 2018;210(2):320–332

Qin S, Caskey CF, Ferrara KW. Ultrasound contrast microbubbles in imaging and therapy: physical principles and engineering. Phys Med Biol 2009;54(6):R27–R57

Webb AG. Introduction to Biomedical Imaging. Wiley; 2002

Zagzebski JA. Essentials of Ultrasound Physics. Mosby; 1996